How To Go (and stay) Vegan

How To Go (and stay) Vegan

Ed Winters

Vermilion
LONDON

VERMILION

UK | USA | Canada | Ireland | Australia
India | New Zealand | South Africa

Vermilion is part of the Penguin Random House group of companies
whose addresses can be found at global.penguinrandomhouse.com

Penguin Random House UK
One Embassy Gardens, 8 Viaduct Gardens, London SW11 7BW

penguin.co.uk
global.penguinrandomhouse.com

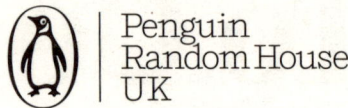

First published by Vermilion in 2025

1

Copyright © Ed Winters 2025

The moral right of the author has been asserted.

Editorial Consultant: Paul Murphy

No part of this book may be used or reproduced in any manner for the purpose of training artificial intelligence technologies or systems. This work is reserved from text and data mining (Article 4(3) Directive (EU) 2019/790).

> The information in this book has been compiled as general guidance on the specific subjects addressed. It is not a substitute and not to be relied on for medical, healthcare or pharmaceutical professional advice. Please consult your GP before changing, stopping or starting any medical treatment. So far as the author is aware the information given is correct and up to date as at September 2025. Practice, laws and regulations all change and the reader should obtain up to date professional advice on any such issues. The author and publishers disclaim, as far as the law allows, any liability arising directly or indirectly from the use or misuse of the information contained in this book.

Typeset in 11/14.6pt Sabon LT Pro by Six Red Marbles UK, Thetford, Norfolk
Printed and bound in Great Britain by Clays Ltd, Elcograf S.p.A.

The authorised representative in the EEA is Penguin Random House Ireland, Morrison Chambers, 32 Nassau Street, Dublin D02 YH68

A CIP catalogue record for this book is available from the British Library

ISBN 9781785045844

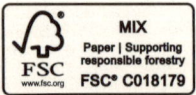

Penguin Random House is committed to a sustainable future for our business, our readers and our planet. This book is made from Forest Stewardship Council® certified paper.

CONTENTS

INTRODUCTION 1

Chapter 1	Why Vegan?	7
Chapter 2	A New Normal	35
Chapter 3	How to Navigate Food	75
Chapter 4	Beyond Food	127
Chapter 5	Now You're Vegan, What Next?	165
Chapter 6	How to Be Vegan in a Non-Vegan World	195
Conclusion		221

Resources 225
Weekly Meal Planner 233
Notes 235
Acknowledgements 247
Index 249
About the Author 259

INTRODUCTION

So, you've seen a documentary, a video or a post online. Or maybe you have a vegan friend or family member who has inspired you. Perhaps you were raised vegetarian, or maybe something just clicked one day. Whatever the reason, you've come to the conclusion that you want to go vegan. The big question now is *how*?

Deciding to become vegan can feel like a daunting task. It does, after all, involve changing many aspects of our lifestyles, including arguably the biggest of all – the food we eat every single day. It's no wonder then that it can feel intimidating to embark on this journey. This becomes even more true if we are doing it on our own, perhaps even against the wishes of our family members or close friends. Add to this that we've most likely met or come across people who say that they tried veganism but it was just 'too hard', or that they felt like they weren't eating healthily. It can all seem so difficult and confusing – what can I eat, what does this label mean, how do I get vitamin B12, and will I have to wear hemp and move to a commune in Portugal?

However, fear not, because you've picked up the right book. What you're reading now is not only going to help you become vegan in the first place, it's going to give you the confidence, tips and knowledge that will help you stay vegan long into the future as well. In essence, it's going to comprehensively break down and answer all of the important questions people have about making the change, ensuring that by the end of the book you have a clear and focused understanding of how to go (and stay) vegan.

This is my third book, but the way I have approached writing it is the same as the two that came before it. *This Is Vegan Propaganda (And Other Lies the Meat Industry Tells You)*, my first, is the book that I wish I'd been given when I was a staunch meat, dairy and egg eater and hadn't really thought about the impact of the choices I was making, and *How to Argue With a Meat Eater (And Win Every Time)* is the one that I wish I'd been given when I first started advocating for veganism. Similarly, with *How to Go (and Stay) Vegan*, I have aimed to write the book that I wish I'd been given more than a decade ago when I decided to go vegan myself, because I too had these questions and worries before I made the change. As such, I would have found this book to be incredibly helpful, because even though I had come to realise that I needed to change my lifestyle, the prospect of actually doing so still felt daunting. However, if I had been able to read this book at that time, it would have made the process of becoming vegan significantly easier for me.

Making the change

When I first went vegan, my best takeaway option was a vegetable pizza without cheese – or, as was the case one time, cheese-less pizza with lettuce on top. I wish I was kidding. My local supermarket didn't exactly cater to vegans either, although I remember feeling like I'd won the jackpot when they started to stock tofu.

When I initially made the change, checking a menu at a restaurant was an exercise in hope more than anything else, and if you could get a vegan option, it was often because you'd asked the kitchen to remove half of the ingredients from the dish. Plus, this was usually after you had politely explained that vegan doesn't mean gluten-free, and, no, vegans don't eat fish – even if it's just a little bit.

Needless to say, a lot has thankfully changed since then. As well as plant-based living becoming more generally accessible and better understood, there has also been a significant rise in awareness around the consequences of what we do to animals and how it impacts them, the planet and us.

That being said, the question of *how* to go vegan is still as important as ever, and the same questions and concerns still remain for many people. This is why I'll be drawing from my own experiences throughout this book, including the mistakes I made and what in hindsight I would do differently. Since making the change, I've dedicated my time to advocating for veganism. I have learned all about the varying issues related to our use of animals, and I have learned extensively about the psychology of behaviour change, the impact of culture and social conditioning on our choices, and, importantly, the challenges that people face when they make the decision to become vegan. In the years that I've been doing this work, I have also met thousands of other vegans, many of whom I have had eye-opening conversations with and whose experiences I have learned so much from. These interactions have also informed the contents of this book, meaning that what is contained in these pages is based on a wide range of knowledge and experience to best equip you to go vegan and thrive.

I will also be exploring the evidence and research on changing habits and addressing all the practical aspects of going vegan, so that this book will provide you with everything that you need to make the process simpler and more achievable, including a list of helpful resources that you can refer to and a template meal plan at the end. Because, let's be honest, it can still be a bit of a minefield at times.

This is precisely why this book goes beyond just food and covers clothing, toiletries, entertainment, socialising, family and more. It addresses important topics such as plant-based alternatives, pets, synthetic leather and raising children on a plant-based diet. Even though things have improved a lot over the years, there's still a lot of misleading discourse around veganism and plant-based diets. The purpose of this book is to cut through the noise and lay everything out in a digestible and helpful way.

Your non-judgemental companion

While veganism is often viewed as the process of giving something up, there is actually so much to be gained from going vegan too. Yes, there are challenges and considerations that come with making the switch, but one thing that can often be overlooked is that it can also be incredibly rewarding and enjoyable. This is one of the core messages of the book, and by reading it, I hope it will not only make the potential challenges more manageable for you, it will also allow you to better embrace and take advantage of all the life-enriching and fulfilling aspects of becoming vegan.

However, it's not just the initial process of going vegan that's important; as previously mentioned, the other aim of this book is to ensure that once you've gone vegan, you stay vegan. This means that it is a resource for you to use and refer back to at any point in your veganism. Annotate it, highlight whatever is most applicable and important to you at any given moment in your life, and reread any sections that are helpful for you in the future. Throughout your transition to veganism and beyond, this book is your non-judgemental companion.

INTRODUCTION

Going vegan is about far more than just changing what we eat and what we wear – it's about aligning our actions with our values and embracing a way of life that has far-reaching and vital benefits. There are many problems in the world, many of which we have no real power over. However, by going vegan we can have a positive impact every single day and derive pride and fulfilment knowing that we are living according to our principles.

As you embark on this important change, the first thing to recognise is that you've already made one of the most important and difficult steps: acknowledging there's a problem and actively seeking out ways you can help be a part of the solution. This means that you have already started the process of going vegan, potentially without even realising it. So keep going, and stay positive and confident in yourself and your capabilities.

One of the most common things that I hear from other vegans, and something that applies to me too, is that going vegan is one of the best decisions they've ever made and that they wish they had done so sooner. It is my hope that by reading and using this book, you too will soon share the same sentiment.

CHAPTER 1

WHY VEGAN?

By virtue of reading this book about how to go vegan, there's a strong chance that you are at least familiar with some the arguments for veganism and a plant-based diet already. That being said, one of the most surprising aspects of veganism is just how many different issues it covers. While you may already have a broad idea of what the problems with animal farming are, one thing I've learned since going vegan is that the issues associated with animal exploitation are far greater than many of us initially realise. Understanding the different problems in more detail is also one of the most important ways of building up commitment and motivation to make the change. For these reasons, it is still worth highlighting the key aspects of veganism, especially if you are on the fence about making the change.

I want to start by covering what veganism actually is, as it can often be misrepresented or misunderstood. I deliberately used both 'veganism' and 'plant-based diet' above, not because a plant-based diet isn't also vegan, but because veganism transcends just diet. In other words, you can eat a plant-based diet and not be vegan. This is because veganism is an ethical belief system that aims to challenge and dismantle animal exploitation in all of its many varied and distinct forms. In fact, in the UK, ethical veganism is protected by law as a philosophical belief.

I mention this because many of you may have picked up this book because you are concerned about the environmental impact of animal farming, or perhaps you are concerned about some of the personal or social health consequences related to animal products. These are all exceptionally important and valid reasons for changing how we live, and I champion them throughout this book, as well as throughout my other books and work more generally.

However, because there can often be confusion around what veganism means and the motivations for going vegan, it can be really helpful to establish the difference between eating plant-based and being vegan. I also strongly believe that connecting with the ethics of what we do to animals is incredibly important, because doing so is a very strong incentive for going and staying vegan.

As mentioned in the introduction, this book is your complete guide to going vegan. It's your one-stop resource when it comes to making the change and succeeding in the long term. However, in order to achieve this, one of the most important factors is to build up your conviction and determination. This way, if you encounter any trickier moments or perhaps slip up and make a mistake, you can bring yourself back to the *why* and gently yet convincingly remind yourself of the reasons you are making the change in the first place.

I also strongly believe that one of the most poorly understood aspects of veganism is how far-reaching and varied its positive consequences are. When I first went vegan, I did so for ethical reasons, driven by a strong feeling that the exploitation of animals violates the moral consideration that should be granted to them. However, since making the change, I have come to realise just how important our choices are in other areas of life too. Animal welfare, the planet, pandemics, antibiotic resistance, chronic disease – the number of things that are positively impacted by one simple choice is truly remarkable.

And it's not that veganism is better for animals but worse for the planet, or that it's better for the planet but increases the risk of pandemics and antibiotic-resistant bacteria – it is beneficial in all of these different regards. And while I would argue that the ethics of what we do to animals is on its own important enough to merit us changing our lifestyles, there is no denying that all of these issues together truly reinforce the urgency of addressing how we view and treat animals.

While realising that there is so much at stake can feel demoralising, it is also empowering to recognise the influence that our decisions actually have. In fact, what we choose to eat is one of the few examples of an everyday decision we can make that can have a profound impact on us and the world at large. Many of us often feel helpless or unable to address the global problems we face, hoping, often in vain, that those in positions of power will step in and fix things. However, while policies and laws have an impact on our food and lifestyle choices, going vegan is one of those rare opportunities where we are not necessarily just reliant on governments or those in positions of authority to create the change we want to see. We can address these issues ourselves by changing how we live, which makes veganism even more appealing and relevant.

Despite the importance and far-reaching consequences of our choices, as a society we do not give them the attention that they deserve. In fact, it's shocking just how unintentional and nonchalant we can be when it comes to deciding what we eat, wear and use. Generally speaking, we eat the food that we do because we enjoy it, because it conforms with the cultural norms of where we live and because we were raised eating it. The food choices we make as adults are consequently choices that are hugely determined by factors related to our environments and upbringing. However, as I will explain in this chapter, these are not the most important factors to consider when it comes to what we eat and consume.

This is why education and awareness are so fundamentally important. First, because they provide us with the knowledge and imperative to change our ways, but also because education is the antidote to ignorance, and action is the antidote to helplessness.

Veganism allows us to feel like we are actively influencing and participating in the world around us, not because we can change everything on our own, but because the choices that we make individually add up to something greater when we group together to form collectives. However, a movement for change is only as strong as all the individuals who are a part of it. Put simply, the choices we make matter. They matter to us. They matter to the planet. They matter to animals.

I mention this because one of the most common arguments I hear from people is that they are just individuals, or that one person making a change won't make a difference. However, if we don't change as individuals, then nothing will change.

It is true that veganism deals with issues and realities that are extremely upsetting or worrying in nature. However, veganism is also about empowerment, both individually and collectively. And, aside from everything else, it's also fun and enjoyable – something that I hope to reinforce throughout the rest of this book.

This change in perspective can be so important when it comes to driving ourselves to make the change, as being faced with the sheer scale of what is wrong can make us feel like our actions are futile or not worthwhile. So even though some of what is discussed below is far from pleasant, informing ourselves about the negative impact of animal consumption can not only make us feel more optimistic, it can also feed our appetite for change. Rather than being a part of the problem, we can instead be a part of the solution.

However, we can only truly grasp all of this if we at least know why the choices we make are so important – and, considering that they have serious ethical, environmental and personal and social health consequences, they certainly are. So let's start with the ethics.

Ethics

The scale of animal exploitation is absolutely massive. For food alone, we slaughter in the region of 85 billion land animals[1] and remove as many as 2.2 trillion fish from our oceans[2] every single year. While these huge numbers are a serious indictment of our exploitation of animals and succinctly show just how large and severe the scale of this problem really is, there is something that can be lost in these numbers: the individuals who make them up.

The problem is that these numbers are so massive that thinking about them is more of an intellectual exercise than an emotional one. After all, how can we empathise with an abstract number? This is why I strongly believe that to connect with the ethics of what we do to animals, it's important to think about the individuals behind these enormous numbers.

For anyone who has lived with a dog or a cat, I'm sure that when you hear about the dog and cat meat trade that exists in certain places around the world, your first thought is to imagine the animal you've lived with in that situation, which is an extremely powerful way of thinking about the problem. Although most of us won't have been raised with or personally exposed to the species of animals that are conventionally exploited, and therefore never had the opportunity to get to know one of them at first hand, connecting the products we purchase with the individuals who have been exploited and harmed is an extremely effective way of understanding the ethical issues around our use and abuse of animals.

Practices that society deems to be perfectly legal allow for animals to be mutilated, forcibly impregnated and kept in cages. They can be macerated alive, shot with bolt guns, electrocuted and forced into gas chambers. Fish are pulled from the oceans and crushed under the weight of one another. They can experience their organs rupturing from the change in pressure and are left to suffocate. And the exploitation is not just limited to food production. Animals are abused in a variety of ways, including having truly chilling experiments performed on them. They can be trapped in aquariums and circuses and forced to perform tricks. Animals used for clothing can be kept in cages and have their feathers plucked and fur pulled off them when they're alive.

Beyond the physical violence, there is also the general undercurrent of subjugation, the lack of autonomy, the feelings of fear, anxiety and terror, and the emotional and psychological suffering that goes along with it. By its very nature, cruelty is an inherent and fundamental part of animal exploitation.

One of the easiest ways of ascertaining whether or not we are more ethically aligned with veganism or animal exploitation is to reflect on what our attitudes towards animals actually are. For example, are we against animal cruelty? If yes, would we consider kicking a dog to be an act of animal cruelty that we would therefore oppose on ethical grounds? Here's the problem: the animals we exploit for food, clothing, entertainment and testing wish that the worst they had to fear was being kicked. Sadly, the experiences that these animals are forced to endure are far worse. Yet what this reveals to us is that we already recognise that what we pay for constitutes animal cruelty – and that we are therefore ethically against it.

When it comes to food, it's not just animals raised specifically for their flesh who are exploited or even slaughtered. In the dairy industry, cows are forcibly impregnated and have their babies taken from them almost immediately after they have been born. This process is the same whether the dairy cows are raised intensively or not. In the egg industry, male chicks are deemed surplus to requirements, so they are macerated alive or gassed to death immediately after being born. The hens are often debeaked before being taken to farms where they can be housed by the thousands in cramped and dirty conditions, a reality for many so-called free-range hens as well. And all egg-laying hens and dairy cows end up in a slaughterhouse when their production of eggs or milk declines.

Some people argue that being a vegetarian is an ethical compromise. However, it's important to remember that the dairy and egg industries are just as unethical as the meat industries, and, in reality, the standard practices that take place on these farms are among the worst on any animal farm.

Even though there are some systems of farming that are less cruel, many of the worst practices still occur in less intensive systems of farming, and the animals still end up in the same slaughterhouses and are killed in the exact same ways. Free-range pigs are still forced into gas chambers. Cattle that graze outside still have their throats cut.

Irrespective of whether or not some systems of animal farming are better, faced with the opportunity not to fund animals being exploited, mutilated, forcibly impregnated or forced into slaughterhouses at all, the fundamental question is: what is the most ethical choice we can make?

I strongly believe that connecting with the ethics of veganism is one of the most important and crucial elements of ensuring that we not only go vegan, but stay vegan. Even if it isn't main the reason you picked up this book or are looking to change how you live, the reality of what we do to animals is incredibly powerful when it comes to finding motivation. This is because it centres the decision around our personal power on the lives of others. Rather than eating animal products being something that only affects us or has an impact that is fairly abstract and not necessarily tangible, thinking about the ethics of animal consumption helps us understand that there are direct victims who are being impacted as a consequence of the choices we are making.

While the feeling of guilt is not a pleasant one, it can be really motivating and push us to make positive changes and empathise with others. However, going vegan isn't about filling ourselves with shame; it's about feeling pride in ourselves by acknowledging the role we play in the lives of others and factoring that into our decision-making.

This feeling of pride in our personal accountability is especially important during the early days of going vegan, when we might have cravings or doubts. It means that in those moments when you might be tempted to buy a piece of steak or order a pizza with mozzarella on it, you can think about the victims of those choices and remind yourself why you are making this change in the first place. Without that strong ethical focus, it can be easier to go back to eating animal products and convince ourselves that just reducing the amount of animal products we eat is enough.

For example, rather than diluting our culpability by thinking that ordering a bucket of chicken is not going to make any significant difference, we can remind ourselves that a bucket of chicken is filled with the bodies of multiple chickens who have lived lives of suffering and have been killed specifically for that serving. That bucket of chicken on its own might not have had a significant impact on the planet, or included chickens infected with bird flu or a strain of resistant bacteria. However, for those chickens in that bucket, our choice means everything.

There are a huge number of exposés and investigation videos available online, and although they are incredibly unpleasant and deeply upsetting to watch, they provide one of the most effective and powerful ways of understanding the true nature of animal exploitation. In the same way that we might imagine our companion animal when we hear about the dog or cat meat trade in another country, watching a video from a farm or slaughterhouse can help us create a visual image next time we are in the meat, dairy or egg aisles. Rather than just seeing the meat, we can bring to mind the individual whose flesh we are looking at. This is why the ethical argument can reshape how we perceive animal products, encouraging us no longer to view them as 'food', in much the same way that we don't consider a dog to be 'food'.

Veganism can get bogged down in politics, social dynamics and misconceptions. Often when this issue is being discussed, it feels like we do not see the wood for the trees. However, if we just boil it down to the fundamentals, when we buy animals products, we are funding the use of contraptions like gas chambers and industrial macerators. We are paying for facilities that exist solely to cut, bleed and kill. The conversation around veganism can be made as complex or as simple as we want it to be, but the bottom line is that causing less fear, suffering, exploitation and slaughter is a good thing.

Antibiotic resistance

It seems hard to believe now, but it wasn't long ago that dying from an infection caused by something as small as a cut was a real possibility. This is because almost all of us alive today have existed in a world where antibiotics have been readily available. As such, the thought of dental work or even a minor cut posing a serious risk to life seems incomprehensible.

However, it would be foolish to take these miracle drugs for granted. The reality is that a post-antibiotic world, in which we have no effective antibiotics left to treat diseases such as typhoid, tuberculosis, meningitis, tetanus and syphilis, or for use in cancer treatments and surgery, among many other lifesaving applications, isn't necessarily just a dystopian science-fiction narrative. The bacteria that antibiotics kill can develop resistance over time, rendering the antibiotics ineffective, and the more antibiotics are used, the higher the risk of bacteria developing resistance to them.

The World Health Organization describes antibiotic resistance as one of the most pressing public-health threats facing humanity, and it is estimated that antimicrobial resistance kills at least 1.2 million people per year, with this number set to increase.[3] It would therefore seem logical that we would prioritise the safeguarding of antibiotics, as they are a vital part of human health. After all, surely something so important wouldn't be used so flippantly?

Sadly, although antibiotics are so important to us humans, it is estimated that globally around 70 per cent of antibiotics are given to farmed animals,[4] highlighting how disproportionate our use of antibiotics for farmed animals is compared to human applications. Because increased antibiotic use is what leads to resistance, the biggest driver of that resistance is therefore animal farming, further emphasising how vital it is that we change how we eat.

Antibiotics are often used routinely, especially in intensive farming systems, where the risk of disease is higher. This means that they are not just used to treat already-infected animals (this is referred to as therapeutic use). If a few animals are found to be sick, all the animals in the group can be given antibiotics to prevent the disease from spreading, even if the vast majority of those animals don't have the disease (this is referred to as metaphylactic use). And antibiotics are also used as a preventative measure even when there are no signs of disease (this is referred to as prophylactic use). Prophylactic use is often carried out en masse by administering the antibiotics to animals via their feed or drinking water. In the case of dairy cows, they can also have antibiotics administered straight into their udders in order to prevent mastitis.

If this weren't bad enough, antibiotics are also used as growth promoters, driving profit rather than as necessary medical interventions. In fact, in the early 1940s, penicillin began to be used experimentally in farmed animals before it had even become widely available to treat humans. Trials showing that low doses of antibiotics led to animals growing faster were carried out in the UK and the USA, and it didn't take long before they were being used rampantly across the animal farming sector. However, rather than being called 'growth promoters', they were given the far more unassuming name of 'digestive enhancers'.

Then, during the 1960s, there were a series of salmonella outbreaks in the UK that hospitalised thousands of people and killed at least four children. The outbreaks were caused by the world's first recorded strain of multidrug-resistant salmonella, which was attributed to the use of antibiotics on farms.[5] Astonishingly, it took until 2006 before the use of antibiotics for growth promotion was banned throughout the EU, and until 2017 for a similar ban to be introduced in the USA. However, the regulations still allow for prophylactic use, which can also have a growth-promoting effect.

Thankfully, across Europe, including in the UK, antibiotic use in farmed animals has decreased since the early 2010s. And in 2022, the EU brought in a new set of regulations to further restrict the use of antibiotics in agriculture, with the UK following suit in 2024. However, unlike the EU, the new UK regulations do not ban prophylactic group treatments or require statutory antibiotic-use data collection.

Besides the fact that antibiotics are still being needlessly used on animal farms in the UK and the EU, antibiotic-resistant bacteria are a global issue – what happens in another country in turn affects us too. This is because resistant bacteria can spread through person-to-person contact as well as through other means such as contaminated foods and surfaces. If the use of antibiotics in farmed animals in other countries leads to the creation and spread of resistant bacteria, these bacteria could then be spread to other areas of the world, including places where there are tighter restrictions around antibiotic use. We urgently need to rethink our antibiotic use worldwide, but instead, despite slow improvements in some areas, the use of antibiotics in farmed animals is actually increasing globally.[6]

It is absurd that we are compromising the miracle of modern medicine to help sustain the morally corrupt and staggeringly inefficient industrial animal farming complex.

And while certain systems of animal farming use antibiotics less, a transition to a plant-based food system is vital if we want to remove antibiotics from our food system as much as possible.

Pandemics

If the threat of antibiotic resistance weren't bad enough, the farming of animals is also a key driver in the emergence and spread of viruses that could cause the next pandemic. While it is true that we can't suppress and avoid all disease outbreaks, it would seem logical that we would at least take the risk of large-scale pandemics seriously and not live in a way that significantly increases the likelihood of them happening. Except by this point we know that what is logical and what is actually happening are not necessarily the same thing. Case in point, animal farming and pandemics.

It is estimated that three out of four emerging infectious diseases in humans originate from animals (known as zoonotic diseases).[7] Throughout history there have been many examples of diseases that have jumped from animals to humans and caused mass deaths and suffering.

According to the United Nations Environment Programme (UNEP), there are seven major human drivers of zoonotic disease emergence.[8] They are:

1) Increasing human demand for animal protein
2) Unsustainable agricultural intensification and in particular domestic livestock farming
3) Increased use and exploitation of wildlife
4) Unsustainable utilisation of natural resources accelerated by urbanisation, land use change and extractive industries
5) Increased travel and transportation

6) Changes in food supply driven by increased demand for animal source food, new markets for wildlife food and agricultural intensification
7) Climate change

The main theme running throughout these seven points is our exploitation of animals. In fact, the UNEP even clarifies that part of the risk with increased travel and transportation is due to the handling and transportation of animals and animal products. And animal farming is also one of the leading drivers of climate change. In other words, every single major human driver of zoonotic disease emergence is either substantially or entirely linked to our exploitation of animals.

When talking about pandemics specifically, the disease that experts fear the most is avian influenza, also known as bird flu. Since the start of the twentieth century, there have been four influenza pandemics, three of them caused by bird flu viruses and the other, in 2009, by a swine flu virus that originated in farmed pigs. The most devastating of these pandemics was in 1918, when between 50 million and 100 million people died, making it potentially the most severe in human history. The virus is believed to have spread to humans from farmed poultry in Kansas.

The issue with farming animals, especially in intensive environments where thousands of them are crammed tightly together, is that they can act as hosts for viruses, allowing the viruses to mutate and spread. If these viruses mutate in such a way as to make them effective at animal-to-human and then human-to-human transmission, we then have the potential for extremely virulent diseases to spread throughout our species. If these viruses have also mutated in a way that makes them deadly, we now have a virus that spreads easily and is effective at killing. When you add in to the mix that the animals we farm are genetically uniform and often stressed, immunocompromised and living in unhygienic conditions, it becomes clear that we are playing with fire when it comes to our farming system.

Our main strategy for combatting viruses when they do arise provides us with a good indication of what our main strategy should be moving forward. Whenever an outbreak of a disease is found on a farm, the animals are culled to prevent further spread. However, if the animals were not there in the first place, the outbreak wouldn't have occurred. So, rather than culling them reactively in the hopes that will stop the spread, we could instead be proactive and not breed them to begin with, thereby ensuring there is no outbreak that needs to be stopped. After all, if we fail to cull the animals in time and stop the spread, the events of the Covid-19 pandemic show us just how quickly viruses can spiral out of control, not to mention the crippling impact they can have socially and economically, let alone the direct loss of life.

However, it's not just the actual farming of animals that increases the risk of spillover events. As will be discussed in more detail in the 'Environment' section of this chapter, animal farming is the leading driver of habitat loss and deforestation. When we turn habitats and wild areas into farmland, we increase the contact we have with wild animals. This is especially important in tropical areas of the world, where disease-carrying wildlife such as mosquitoes, bats and rodents, among others, are more commonly found. However, it is these areas that are currently being deforested the most, with the leading driver of that deforestation being animal farming. By encroaching into wild areas and then farming domesticated animals in them, we are introducing a continuous supply of animals who are now in closer contact with disease-carrying wild animals and who can act as potential hosts for viruses to mutate within. We then take these animals and drive them to different farms, as well as slaughterhouses, meat markets and other populated areas where these viruses have direct contact with humans. This is how viruses such as Nipah and SARS moved from animals to humans.

In addition to this, as climate change renders increasing areas of previously farmable land infertile, people may resort to eating more wild animals, including bushmeat. Ebola and HIV, two of the most devastating infectious diseases to date, are both believed to have originated from bushmeat consumption. There are also food-borne pathogens like E. coli, salmonella and campylobacter, which infect hundreds of millions of people every year, and which we could significantly reduce the prevalence of if we stopped farming and eating animals.

We will never be able to fully safeguard ourselves against infectious diseases or completely eliminate the risk of spillover events. However, our current systems of animal exploitation are maximising the chances of more pandemics, epidemics and infectious diseases occurring. Animal exploitation might not be the only risk factor, but it is by far the largest. This is why if we ever want to minimise as far as we can the risk of infectious diseases and pandemics, addressing our use and abuse of animals has to be front and centre.

Chronic disease

In later chapters, I will discuss how to make sure you're eating a healthy plant-based diet, covering topics such as nutrients and supplements. However, one of the many positive consequences of eating a wholefoods plant-based diet is that it can help us live healthier and longer lives, with a reduced risk of developing many of the most common chronic diseases. One of the key reasons for this is that by removing foods that have been shown to increase chronic disease risk – particularly red meat and processed meat – we have the opportunity to increase our daily intake of foods that have been shown to decrease chronic disease risk, such as legumes, wholegrains, fruits and vegetables.

In other words, plant-based diets are not just beneficial because we are removing foods that can cause negative health outcomes, but also because they encourage us to eat more foods that promote positive health outcomes. It's essentially a win-win. For example, the largest study to date analysing the link between meat consumption and diabetes showed that processed meat, unprocessed red meat and poultry were all associated with an increased risk of developing type 2 diabetes,[9] while other studies have shown that plant-based diets are associated with a lower risk of developing type 2 diabetes.[10]

In regards to heart disease, the largest review of all large-scale studies to date looking at meat and heart disease showed that consumption of processed meat and red meat increased the risk of coronary heart disease.[11] At the same time, studies have shown that plant-based diets are associated with a lower risk of heart disease.[12]

The same is true of cancer, with the World Health Organization's International Agency for Research on Cancer classifying processed meat as a class 1 carcinogen and unprocessed red meat as a class 2 carcinogen. Since these classifications, even more evidence has been published showing that meat is associated with an increased risk of cancer, particularly gastrointestinal cancer.[13] At the same time, studies have shown that plant-based diets are associated with a reduced risk of cancer.[14]

These chronic illnesses are particularly relevant, as cardiovascular diseases are the biggest killer of both men and women globally,[15] type 2 diabetes is one of the most common chronic diseases in the world, with its prevalence increasing, and bowel cancer is the second most common cause of cancer death globally,[16] with only lung cancer killing more people.[17]

This ever-growing body of evidence is leading to changes in nutrition guidelines, with leading health authorities in countries including the UK, Denmark, Germany and Canada, among others, all shifting towards advocating for more plant-foods and fewer animal-derived foods.

In fact, an umbrella review, which assessed 48 other systematic reviews published between January 2000 and June 2023, found that plant-based diets are 'significantly associated' with better health markers overall. These include lower cholesterol, better regulation of blood sugar levels, healthier body weight, less inflammation and lower risk of heart disease and cancer.[18]

This isn't just a positive in terms of personal health, but it also helps when it comes to protecting healthcare systems and reducing the cost implications of healthcare provision. The less money is spent on preventable diseases, the more money can be used to improve services and treat patients. This is especially important as the global population continues to grow. For example, a study analysing the impact of diet shifts on global health found that swapping to plant-based diets would lead to millions fewer deaths per year, alongside health-related cost savings of around 1 trillion US dollars annually.[19]

It's important to note that a healthy lifestyle goes beyond diet alone, and we can't eliminate the risk of chronic diseases entirely. However, it's empowering to know that adopting a vegan lifestyle at least minimises the risks and allows us to take more control over our health and lives.

Environment

The sustainability of our food system is becoming more important by the day. Our population is increasing, while at the same time climate change and the degradation of our natural world poses an ever-growing risk to food security. As a consequence, transforming our food system is essential if want to ensure that everyone has access to a nutritious and sustainable diet.

The problem is, although our food system is changing, it's not changing for the better. Global meat demand has quadrupled since 1961 and continues to grow.[20] All of this has led to serious environmental problems and has caused our food system to be become untenable.

So, to understand the impact that animal farming has, let's break it down into the key issues.

EMISSIONS

Just as with other sectors, greenhouse gas emissions are an essential part of the conversation when it comes to farming and sustainability. This is because food is responsible for around 25–30 per cent of global emissions,[21] and animal farming is conservatively responsible for 14.5 per cent of global annual greenhouse gas emissions, which is nearly six times more than the entire aviation industry.[22] If things continue as they are, the emissions from food alone will push the global average temperature past 1.5°C and even as far as 2°C by the end of the twenty-first century.[23] In other words, changing how we eat is essential if we want to avoid climate catastrophe.

While the conversation around greenhouse gas emissions often centres around carbon dioxide, methane and nitrous oxide are also a crucial part of agriculture's impact. Methane is so important that the executive director of UNEP stated that 'cutting methane is the strongest lever we have to slow climate change over the next 25 years and complements necessary efforts to reduce carbon dioxide'.[24]

Methane has a higher global-warming potential than carbon dioxide, which means that per equivalent mass, methane is more effective at trapping heat. In fact, to date, only carbon dioxide has contributed more to global warming than methane. So how does this relate to animal farming? Well, agriculture is the biggest emitter of methane globally,[25] with 80 per cent of that coming specifically from animal farming.[26] Methane is produced by the digestive systems of ruminant animals (a process known as enteric fermentation), and it can also be released from animal manure.

The good news is that methane also breaks down in around 12 years, meaning that it is only in the atmosphere for a relatively short period of time. With animal farming being the single biggest source of methane emissions, going plant-based is therefore one of the most effective things that we can do to slow climate change.

But it's not just methane. Agriculture produces around 80 per cent of nitrous oxide emissions.[27] This greenhouse gas is produced by microbes in soil that convert nitrogen from fertilisers, animal urine and animal manure into nitrous oxide. Over a 100-year time span, nitrous oxide has a global-warming potential nearly 300 times that of carbon dioxide,[28] and it is the third most important greenhouse gas after carbon dioxide and methane. By eliminating animal farming, we can reduce the amount of land being used to grow food, meaning that we can reduce the amount of fertiliser being used. It would also remove the copious amounts of urine and manure that animals produce too.

LAND USE

Almost half of the world's total habitable land is used for agriculture. Of that, around 80 per cent is used for animal farming, with only 16 per cent used to grow crops directly for human consumption.[29] This means that animal farming is the single biggest user of land globally. Despite this, animal products only provide 17 per cent of the calories and 37 per cent of the protein consumed globally.[30] This means that growing plants for human consumption is far more efficient, as it allows us to produce more food and nutrition while using significantly less land.

But why is using less land for farming so important in the first place?

No industry has caused greater or more harmful transformation of the planet's wild terrestrial habitats and ecosystems than animal farming. Converting that land into agricultural land suitable for grazing or growing feed crops is the single biggest driver of deforestation and habitat and biodiversity loss.[31] Cattle ranching alone is the biggest driver of deforestation in Brazil, with studies showing it is responsible for around three-quarters of deforestation in the region.[32]

However, this is not just an issue in South America. The use of land for animal farming and resulting biodiversity loss is a problem across the USA, the EU and the UK. In fact, around 85 per cent of agricultural land in the UK is used for animal farming,[33] which is equal to just under half of the entire landmass of Great Britain and Northern Ireland.[34] Shockingly, the UK ranks in the bottom 10 per cent of countries in the world when it comes to biodiversity intactness.[35]

Land use change isn't just bad when it comes to biodiversity loss. Deforestation and soil degradation also cause greenhouse gas emissions, as they lead to carbon being emitted.

So how does being vegan help?

We have already established that producing plants directly for human consumption is more efficient than grazing animals or growing crops to feed to animals. This means that the more plants and the fewer animal products we consume, the less land will be needed to produce food. In fact, if the world swapped to a plant-based food system, we would be able to feed every mouth on the planet and reduce the amount of agricultural land by 75 per cent.[36] Put into perspective, this is an area of land equivalent in size to Australia, China, the EU and the USA combined no longer being needed to produce food.

Because we've already established that animal farming is the biggest driver of deforestation and biodiversity loss, removing animal farming could instead be the biggest driver of reforestation and biodiversity gains. We could rewild these areas of land, allowing us to sequester carbon by harnessing the power of photosynthesis, which plants use to grow and build up their organic biomass. This is why reducing methane 'complements necessary efforts to reduce carbon dioxide' – because removing animals from our food system not only means reducing methane, it also allows us to maximise the potential of drawing down and storing carbon as well.

FISHING

When discussing food and the environment, fish are often considered to be an environmentally friendly choice, but is this true?

When compared to other animal products – such as beef, lamb and dairy – fish and marine animals do tend to have a lower carbon footprint, although certain farmed and wild marine animals – such as wild lobster, wild shrimp, farmed shrimp and wild bivalves – can have a higher carbon footprint than chickens.[37] However, the lower carbon footprint associated with fish and marine animals overall doesn't take into account the sustainability of wild fish stocks. Even if consuming one species of fish results in fewer greenhouse gas emissions than consuming another, if that fish came from a fishery where the number of fish is in decline, that would mean it was unsustainable regardless of the emissions.

What we deem to be sustainable becomes an even more pertinent question when we consider the role of blue carbon, which is a term used to describe carbon dioxide that is stored in coastal and marine ecosystems. The oceans are the planet's largest carbon sink and have been referred to by the United Nations as 'the world's greatest ally against climate change'.[38] For example, marine habitats such as seagrasses and mangroves can sequester carbon dioxide from the atmosphere at up to four times the rate that terrestrial forests can.[39]

Carbon is also sequestered in the ocean by marine phytoplankton and is then transferred into marine animals through the food chain. When terrestrial organisms die, the carbon contained within them is typically released into the atmosphere. However, when marine animals die, they often sink and the carbon contained within them can be stored at the bottom of the oceans. Simply put, the more animals in the oceans, the more carbon that is stored. However, when we remove marine animals from our oceans, we disrupt the carbon cycle and limit carbon storage. This means that fisheries prevent blue carbon sequestration.[40]

This brings us back to the concept of sustainable fishing. When fisheries are operating at what the fishing industry calls maximum sustainable yield, this doesn't mean that the number of fish in those fisheries is at the highest number it can be. In fact, the growth rates of wild animal populations are often greatest when the overall population size is moderate. This means that fisheries typically keep fish levels at somewhere around 37–50 per cent of what they were pre-fishing.[41] This system of fishery maintenance might maximise the number of fish that can be removed without jeopardising the actual existence of the fish species, but it also means the fishing industry is actively working to keep fish biomass at a lower level.

Aquaculture, which is the farming of marine animals, is now a larger source of seafood than wild fisheries. However, these systems of farming also have sustainability concerns, including water pollution, where nutrient build-up can cause algal blooms and harm aquatic life. Aquaculture can also be responsible for habitat loss, in both coastal and terrestrial areas. Because these farms are factory farms for fish, diseases are rampant, leading to antibiotic use and disease outbreaks, which can lead to infectious diseases, sea lice and parasites being spread to wild populations of marine animals.

Farmed fish also require feed, which can come from wild-caught fish, meaning the sustainability impacts of wild fisheries can also be applicable in the case of farmed fish too. For non-carnivorous animals, plant-based feed can be used. However, growing crops to feed farmed fish contributes to the sustainability issues associated with feed production, and it also creates inefficiency, as those crops could be grown for human consumption instead.

Put simply, regardless of whether certain marine animals are more sustainable than certain terrestrial animals, eating plants over marine animals is still the most sustainable choice. Plus, in the same way that no longer eating terrestrial animals provides us with the best opportunity for storing carbon in our terrestrial ecosystems and increasing terrestrial biodiversity, not eating marine animals provides us with the best opportunity to do the same in our marine ecosystems.

Our choices matter

This conversation about the environmental impact of animal farming and fishing is especially important in high-income nations, as these are the places where per capita animal product consumption tends to be the greatest. This means that the choices those of us who live in the West make are especially important, as our impact is disproportionately higher per capita than the global average. A study that analysed the real diets of 55,000 people in the UK showed that a plant-based diet would result in 75 per cent less greenhouse gas emissions, water pollution and land use, and 54 per cent less water use.[42]

Research is so important when it comes to inspiring ourselves and recognising the hugely positive impact that our choices are having. Seeing that plant-based diets are substantially better in such a wide variety of ways is a really great way of feeling empowered about going vegan, and it can also serve as an important factor when it comes to staying vegan.

Some people who are concerned about the climate impact of their diets choose animal products with a lower climate impact. This leads to people choosing to eat more fish and chickens. However, not only do these animals often live worse lives or experience crueller deaths, the number of animals killed to acquire the same number of calories is far higher. This means that there is a direct trade-off, with more sustainable meat options often being less ethical. However, there is no trade-off when it comes to choosing a plant-based diet, as it is both the most sustainable and the most ethical option available.

Knowledge is power

Like I mentioned at the start of this chapter, there is a good chance that you probably already knew at least some of what I have just covered. However, I hope that laying out some of the key issues has reaffirmed to you why you have picked up this book and why you want to go vegan. Often people make the decision to go vegan without necessarily fully understanding all of the merits of that decision. But knowledge is power, and the more informed we are, the more drive and motivation we can then invest in going and staying vegan.

One of the biggest difficulties in going vegan is processing the magnitude of the mistreatment and remaining optimistic. It can be hard to come to terms with the severity of animal exploitation and how ubiquitous it is (more on this in Chapter 6). As a result, it's understandable that you might become vegan and then try not to think too much about the problems that exist. After all, it's not healthy or advisable to spend every day getting progressively more upset about all the issues that we face in the world. That being said, it's important to maintain a sense of balance and to reaffirm to ourselves why we have made the changes that we have. This is why it is important to reframe our perspective. So, instead of viewing all of these problems just from the perspective of how terrible they are, we can also focus on the fact that we are a part of the solution. This broader sense of empowerment is an extremely useful way of feeling motivated by the problems we are addressing, as opposed to being demotivated by the scale and severity of them.

Change can be slow, and it's not always a straight line. Nonetheless, the importance of that change remains. Instead of feeling swamped by the magnitude of the problems, we should instead feel pride in ourselves for doing something about them.

So, now that we've explored the *why*, let's delve into the *how*.

CHAPTER 2

A NEW NORMAL

Understanding behaviour change and veganism

Now that we've discussed the reasons why it's important to change, the next step is to understand the nature of building habits and creating a new normal. Changing behaviours is notoriously one of the most challenging things that we can do. Even with the best intentions in the world, being tempted or struggling to overcome the difficulties associated with behaviour change can quickly derail us and lead to us ending up back where we started – albeit now feeling more disappointed and frustrated with ourselves.

The process of behaviour change can also vary between people. For some, it can be as easy as deciding something and then simply doing it, whereas for others there might be more challenges and obstacles. Many people underestimate what is required or are not prepared enough going into the change. And when we consider that our brains can fall foul of cognitive biases like status quo bias (finding comfort in maintaining what we have grown used to and therefore trying to avoid the discomfort of change and uncertainty), we can begin to see how our brains are often hardwired in such a way as to oppose behaviour change.

Deconstructing behaviour change and exploring it through a more rational and objective lens helps us take out some of the emotional element and normalises the process, including some of the challenges. This means we can have more self-empathy and understanding. This is especially important in an age where we are bombarded with people masquerading as self-help gurus and motivational speakers, and where social media is filled with people sharing anecdotes about how they've transformed their life or gone from broke to wealthy in the span of 12 months, all of which can lead to us feeling ashamed and confused as to why we keep struggling.

Yet the simple truth is behaviour change can be difficult. This is why it's important to analyse how we build a new normal before we actually dive into the practical aspects of what being a vegan involves.

So, what are some key considerations and techniques that you can use to make going and staying vegan feel less daunting, more exciting and ultimately more successful?

A NEW HABIT

The change to veganism isn't just about incorporating a new habit; it's also about disrupting a current one. However, the behaviour we are disrupting is one that most of us have engaged in our whole lives, and one that many of us have probably taken a fair amount of enjoyment from. Not only that, it's a communal behaviour – it's something that we share with others and form memories around, and it makes up a significant part of our cultures, traditions and festivities.

On the other hand, the new habit is one that is often perceived as inconvenient, requiring willpower and reducing the enjoyment we get from food. Looked at like this, it's easy to see why this change can be perceived to be hard and why it can lead to recidivism. The one thing that veganism does have on its side, though, is the reasons why it is so important. Unlike behaviour changes such as wanting to exercise more, drink more water or eat healthier, which are individual actions that we undertake on our own behalf, veganism represents a change that isn't just for our own personal betterment.

However, it's also important to approach veganism from a positive perspective, framing our decision as something that makes us happy, enthusiastic and empowered. Rather than somewhat begrudgingly making the change because our ethics and values determine that we need to, we can instead celebrate the fact that aligning our ethics, values and actions together is actually an incredibly rewarding and positive experience. And rather than viewing veganism from the perspective of what we are 'giving up' or 'going to miss', we can instead think about it from the perspective of what we are going to gain. Some of those gains are physical, such as the opportunity to cook new foods and have different experiences, but others are emotional – these can include a sense of pride and a sense of purpose. After all, it can make us feel emotionally good to be able to positively reflect on our actions.

Going vegan can also foster a sense of belief in our own capabilities more generally. This is because making a change, especially one with the significance that veganism represents, can instil a sense of confidence in ourselves and what we can achieve. Perhaps we want to incorporate more changes into our life, or we want to learn something new or overcome some obstacle or challenges – having achieved a change previously can offer us a strong sense of self-belief that can permeate other areas of our lives as well. So, as well as veganism having the potential to improve our physical wellbeing, it can provide us with a greater sense of emotional and psychological wellbeing too.

RESHAPING OUR PERSPECTIVE

Even changing how we phrase things can be surprisingly effective. Sometimes as vegans we might say, 'I can't eat that,' but that's not actually accurate. We could eat something animal-based, but instead we *choose* not to. The understanding that what we are doing is a choice is important for several reasons.

First, when we feel like we *have* to do something, it can make us feel restricted or as if we lack autonomy, reducing our desire to act. The understanding that it's a choice can make any initial cravings easier to deal with too. Thinking to ourselves, *I wish I could eat some steak*, or, *I can't eat that cheese*, can make us feel envious, resentful or frustrated. So framing our decision as a choice can make us feel more in control and more accepting of those initial cravings. You *could* eat a piece of steak, you *could* eat some cheese, but you *choose* not to because of what that choice involves.

I reference this due to my own personal experience. When I first stopped eating animals, I went to the house of a friend who was cooking steak. In response to the red meat they were cooking, I said, 'I wish I could eat that too,' which not only created a negative impression of veganism to my friend, who will have viewed my choice to go vegan as a form of deprivation and sacrifice, but misrepresented the situation. I could have chosen to eat the steak, but I didn't. While I might have been craving some steak in that moment, and having an internal conflict about whether or not I could justify having some, I also made the situation harder for myself by phrasing my choice as something that was going against my wishes when this wasn't actually the case.

In a similar way, you could kick a dog without anyone ever knowing and without facing any social repercussions. But the reason you don't is not because you *can't*, it's because you *choose* not to. The reason for this choice is because you understand that it's wrong and doing so would make you feel guilty.

Sometimes we perceive guilt as being a purely negative emotion, but guilt can actually be extremely positive because of what it can teach us about our true feelings. When you consider what happens to animals, you might feel guilty that you have been a part of that system of exploitation. That feeling of guilt shows that you have empathy and that you care, which therefore encourages you to abstain from contributing to that system any longer. I'll revisit this idea later in this chapter.

Another way of reshaping your perspective is to challenge your view of animal products as food. When we consider all of the animals and animal secretions we could eat, it's actually remarkable how few we view as food. Many of us wouldn't consider eating cat or dolphin meat, or drinking rats' or dogs' milk. This would be true even if such products were offered to us. This is because we don't think of these products as *food*.

It's also interesting to imagine how people would react if, in a supermarket, they had the choice between a bottle of human breast milk or a bottle of cow udder milk. Considering we were initially raised on human milk, and it is meant for humans, while cows' milk is meant for calves, from an objective position it would seem more rational to view the human milk as being more acceptable for human consumption. Yet, due to cultural norms, and because we are weaned off human milk and onto cows' milk, from an edibility perspective there's a high chance people would opt for the cows' milk over the human milk.

This is why perception is so crucial, as the way we view different animal products determines how we engage with them. Next time you're in the supermarket and you're looking at a piece of meat, try to imagine it came from a different species of animal. If that was a piece of horse or guinea pig flesh, how would that make you feel? Would you still think of the piece of meat as being food, or would you instead see the meat and think of the horse or guinea pig that the flesh used to be a part of?

CONNECTING THE DOTS

The previous thought experiment touches on a wider point, which is that a really effective way of changing our perception is to be more conscious and connected to the animal products that are available to us. The language we use to describe animal products and the fact that animal farming is out of sight and out of mind means that the supply chain is set up in such a way as to optimise unconscious and disconnected consumption. In addition, the advertising and marketing around animal products also serve to obfuscate the truth and create a vision of animal farming that fails to truthfully represent the reality of animal exploitation and its consequences. This is why being more deliberate and more conscious in our choices is so important.

One way to do this is to connect the animal products with the animals and the harm that preceded that product arriving in the supermarket. Before I stopped eating animals, I used to love the taste of steak. For me, when I saw a piece of steak, I viewed that steak from the perspective of my own personal enjoyment – I didn't think about a cow in a slaughterhouse. I approached purchasing steak from a position of disconnection. To me steak was just a food, and a particularly tasty food at that. However, what helped me initially when I stopped eating red meat was broadening my perspective of a piece of steak beyond the enjoyable sensory experience it offered me and instead considering the horrific sensory experiences that were endured by the animal. This broader perspective was what encouraged me not to eat steak when I was at my friend's house in that anecdote I previously referenced.

Don't worry if this doesn't come naturally at first – we've spent our whole lives eating animal products and associating certain animals with food. Even if we have emotionally and intellectually acknowledged that we want to go vegan, we're still challenging and changing our lifelong mindsets and perceptions, and this can take time.

You don't need to ignore or repress the fact that you have enjoyed these products in the past, nor does it mean feeling shame or feeling negatively about yourself because you have historically enjoyed how they taste. It's about establishing a more connected, well-rounded and balanced perspective today, as a result of which you can make more rational choices that are better reflective of your values and ethics.

So, if you find yourself craving an animal product, standing in front of the cheese aisle in a supermarket or reading about a meat dish on a restaurant menu, it can be really valuable to just pause and take a moment to reflect on those products. Who did they come from? What happened to them? Do these products align with your values? If you purchased and ate them, how would you feel afterwards?

Although I haven't forgotten that I used to enjoy the taste of steak, I no longer view it as a food item that I want to consume. My perspective has changed, and now when I see steak I think of it as cow flesh. This also touches on another means of reshaping our view of animal products. Instead of thinking of animals as meat, it can be powerful to change the terminology and refer to it as 'flesh'. For example, instead of using the word 'bacon', you can call it 'pig flesh'.

The animal farming industry often uses words to minimise the severity of what it does, such as referring to slaughter as 'processing'. We can turn this on its head and use language to emphasise the severity of what happens to animals, and in doing so challenge and update our pre-existing perception of these animal products.

Another alternative to saying 'I don't eat meat' is to instead say, 'I don't eat animals.' This phrasing can be subtly powerful when you use it in front of people. Even though we intellectually and rationally know that meat comes from animals, we often don't consciously make the association. However, if we say to people, 'I don't eat animals,' not only does this reinforce the shift in our own perspective, it also reframes the conversation around meat consumption and encourages other people to more directly connect meat with animals in their own lives too.

GRADUAL ADAPTATIONS

While our tastebuds are normally perceived as being one of the things that make going vegan more challenging, the way they work can actually mean that they ultimately end up helping us.

For many of us, the foods we enjoyed as children are not the same as the foods we enjoy today. When I was a child, I had a strong dislike of mushrooms, but I very much enjoy them now. This is because our tastebuds change over time, meaning that we can adapt to new flavour profiles. This can be seen with how we process salty or sweet food. A study analysing people on a reduced-sugar diet found that during the second month on the diet, the people eating less sugar perceived a low-sugar pudding as being sweeter than the people who hadn't changed their sugar intake.[1] This suggests that changing our eating habits can alter how we perceive the flavour of different foods. People who grow accustomed to eating spicy food often refer to non-spicy food as bland, yet foods that aren't spicy can still be full of flavour. If someone who found non-spicy food bland was to cut out spice from their diet, over time they would begin to find non-spicy food more enjoyable and flavoursome.

Something similar can happen when you go vegan. Over time, plant-foods can become more enjoyable, and the appeal of animal products can lessen. For example, while I was never someone who enjoyed drinking a glass of cows' milk on its own, I did enjoy having cows' milk in tea, coffee and on cereal. Nowadays, as well as having an ethical aversion to cows' milk, I also have a strong aversion to the smell of it in coffee too. On the occasions when I've been accidentally given a coffee made with cows' milk rather than a plant-based milk, I find the taste really strong and unpleasant – but I didn't used to feel that way.

So it's not just that our psychological perception of these foods can change; our sensorial perceptions can change as well.

BE PREPARED

Challenging how we view animal products can be extremely helpful. However, the bedrock of successful behaviour change is being prepared. But what exactly does that involve when it comes to going vegan?

The first stage of becoming prepared relates to what we've already discussed: becoming motivated and informed about all the reasons why you want to make the change. Maintaining a focus on all of those reasons will help you stay on track and will keep reminding you why you have gone vegan in the first place.

However, once we feel informed, the next stage is to put a plan in place so that we can make the change and give ourselves the best possible start. This involves thinking about ways to maximise our chances of succeeding, as well as identifying what could be some of the potential difficulties we will face. If we can foresee any potential challenges, it means we can find ways to minimise the impact that they could have. For example, is there a specific food you think you'll struggle to cut out the most? Do you think you'll find the social aspects harder? Or do you think you'll struggle more when you're at home cooking for yourself?

I'll talk more specifically about recipes, nutrients and food in Chapter 3. However, part of becoming prepared includes thinking about what food we will eat. A really easy way to do this is to have a selection of simple and easy recipes lined up in advance. A good way of approaching this is to think about what meals you already like to eat and work out if you can simply make those meals plant-based. Just changing one or two ingredients can often make a dish vegan. For example, with pasta it could be as easy as swapping any animal protein with a plant protein and then using a vegan alternative for the parmesan. If you make curries, you could instead use a vegan yoghurt or cream and then swap any animal protein for a plant protein.

So rather than going vegan and then thinking to yourself, *What on earth do I eat now?* get ahead of yourself and have some recipes lined up in advance. This also means that you can avoid getting home and realising you don't know what you're cooking, and opening the cupboards only to see empty shelves staring back at you. One simple tip is to create a meal plan (such as the one in the back of this book); that way you know ahead of time what you are going to be eating. Another advantage of having recipes lined up is that you can get the ingredients in advance. This means you can take away the stress of having to buy food after you've had a busy day.

This goes beyond just the food aspects. Informing yourself in advance about what supplements you should start taking, as well as which personal hygiene products are suitable for vegans, makes incorporating all of these different elements of living vegan far easier and more manageable (and I cover both in later chapters). The hardest part of going vegan is right at the beginning, so being prepared is about setting yourself up in such a way as to make the initial change as easy and simple as possible.

HUNGER AND BEHAVIOUR

Another aspect of being prepared is understanding that the pursuit of food is one of the strongest drivers of our behaviour and emotions. This makes perfect sense – we need to eat to stay alive, so the feeling of hunger is an essential part of human survival. However, in a modern world where food is more readily available, the feeling of hunger can sometimes be unhelpful. For example, being hungry can make us irritable, impatient, reactive and impulsive. It can also make our minds wander and allow us to become fixated on what we want to eat, which isn't necessarily the same as what we would choose to eat if we were being less driven by emotion. Case in point: it's why the decisions we make in a supermarket when we're hungry are not necessarily the same decisions we would make if we had just eaten.

This is especially important to consider when talking about the initial transition to veganism, as our hunger could very likely cause us to start craving the foods we used to enjoy. If you combine this with the fact that our actions are then also being driven by a more emotional and impulsive state, it becomes easy to see how we might give in to temptation, even if that goes against what we rationally want. We've all been in a situation where we've ordered or bought something because we're really hungry, only to regret it afterwards.

So, being aware of how hunger can negatively influence us is really important when shaping our new normal. This brings me back to the idea of thinking tactically, such as by creating a meal plan, or by making sure that you have food available and that you're eating enough to feel satisfied. If you're someone who likes to graze, having some plant-based snacks to eat throughout the day can also be really helpful. Snacking is often associated with unhealthy foods, so you could also use going vegan as an opportunity to incorporate healthier foods into your diet. For example, you could opt for nuts, fruit, edamame or vegetables with a vegan dip. Alternatively, you could roast some chickpeas in advance and have those instead of a bag of crisps. That being said, crisps are my personal kryptonite snack, and being vegan doesn't mean that we can't enjoy an unhealthy treat. However, even non-meat-flavoured crisps can contain ingredients like milk powder, so make sure you double-check that the flavours you like are suitable for vegans.

Another tip is to make your food choices before you're hungry. For example, if you tend to grab lunch when you are out and about, you could take some time to research where you can get a plant-based lunch. That way you're not going to be wandering around hungry and potentially in a rush.

WHAT ABOUT CRAVINGS?

However, even if you are prepared, you might still end up craving some of the foods that you used to eat. The first thing to recognise is that having cravings is completely to be expected, as there's a very good chance that by going vegan you are abstaining from eating foods that you enjoyed. So, if you do develop a craving or find yourself thinking about eating something animal-based, take the emotion out of it and just view it for what it is. You're not a bad person for having a craving, nor does a craving mean that you lack the ability to commit to being vegan. A craving arises simply as a consequence of you thinking about something that you used to enjoy. If we can view any temptation from a more objective position, it not only makes it easier for us to understand, it also takes away some of the worry or trepidation that can arise if we start overanalysing or worrying about it.

There is a difference between guilt and shame. For some people, making the change will be more straightforward than it is for others. I've met vegans who went from meat eater to vegan overnight and never looked back. I've also met vegans who found it more challenging in the beginning and either made some mistakes or even relapsed for a period of time. But there isn't a vegan hierarchy where people who went vegan overnight and never had any problems are 'more vegan' or 'better vegans'. There is no shame in making a mistake. The whole point of this book, and about going vegan in general, is that it's not just about the next four weeks; it's about where you'll be in four years and beyond.

This doesn't mean that you should approach becoming vegan with the view that you *will* slip up or that it's OK to order a cow burger one evening. Instead, resolve to do your best and have a plan of action for if you do give in to temptation. As with all things, it's important to hope for the best and plan for the worst.

Change is about establishing a balance between understanding and accountability. It's imperative that we understand the difficulties related to changing behaviours and have compassion for ourselves during that process. However, it's also imperative that we keep pushing ourselves and striving to do our best.

If you do give in to a craving and slip up, the important thing is that you just keep going. What you want to avoid is having a complete relapse where you go back to living the way you did before. This brings us back to guilt and shame. If you slip up and then feel guilty about the mistake, that's an important feeling to hold on to and reflect upon. The guilt in that case is showing you that you don't want to slip up. However, slipping up doesn't make you a bad person, and it doesn't mean that you should chastise yourself for doing so. Shaming yourself is not an effective way of creating a positive outcome – in fact, it does the opposite. It demotivates you and fills your head with negativity, including about the change itself. If you associate going vegan with these punishing and negative thoughts, you are creating an impression that links going vegan with something ultimately undesirable and even detrimental to your overall wellbeing and perception of yourself.

Shaming often goes hand in hand with making sweeping and inaccurate generalisations about ourselves, also known as selective abstractions, which are a type of cognitive bias whereby we focus on a small detail while overlooking the larger context. It can mean that we end up concentrating our energy on a negative and ignoring any positives. So, if you're vegan for two weeks and then slip up, you might think to yourself that you've 'ruined your veganism' or that you've 'undone everything you'd managed over the past two weeks'. This would be a selective abstraction.

You might have made a mistake, but invalidating everything based on that mistake overlooks the fact that for two weeks you've been living vegan. That's a huge positive that provides much-needed context and reassurance. You shouldn't ignore the mistake, but you also shouldn't allow it to completely distort or negatively colour the entirety of what you have achieved so far.

So, instead of attacking yourself for any mistakes, try to view the situation more objectively. You've made a mistake, it's not the end of the world, and it doesn't mean that all of your efforts have been for nothing or that you can't now just continue where you left off. A mistake does not define your ability to change, nor does it reflect poorly on you as a person.

What you don't want to do is view going vegan as being too hard and revert to eating animal products as you did before. Overly negative, self-punishing thoughts can create the impression that the task in front of you is one that you are not able to accomplish – which is not true. In fact, a mistake is an opportunity to learn. It prompts us to work out what went wrong and how to avoid it happening again in the future. So, rather than viewing a setback as an obstacle to you changing, you can instead view it as part of the process of change.

The same is also true even if you have more of a full-blown relapse and go back to eating animal products. If you do end up relapsing, it's important to try and regain a sense of objectivity. Can you establish a sense of control over your actions and pay attention to your thoughts and feelings? Take a moment to reflect on what caused the relapse. This means that rather than perceiving a slip-up or relapse as something that is only negative, it can instead be viewed as an opportunity to improve and understand more about our own behaviour.

It's important to bear in mind that you're not a different person to the one you were when you decided to go vegan in the first place. You probably feel just as strongly about it now; it's just that you've become disconnected from those reasons. So all you need to do is simply, and gently, remind yourself of why you wanted to make the change to begin with.

Reread the first chapter of this book, watch some footage of what happens to animals, sit and take the time to contemplate the consequences of eating animal products. From that point you can then reaffirm to yourself why you wanted to make the change and begin the process of going vegan again. However, this time around you'll be more experienced, have a greater understanding of what is involved and, importantly, be able to learn from your previous mistakes and put a plan in place so that you can hopefully avoid relapsing again.

I have often heard from people who tried to go vegan but went back that it was just 'too hard' for them, while others say that they just don't have the discipline or ability to do it. However, this is not the case. This is why I strongly believe that it's important to take it day by day at the beginning. It can be extremely daunting going into a big change and thinking, *This is it for the rest of my life.* So, rather than viewing going vegan from the perspective of it being a lifelong commitment, just make the commitment that the next meal will be plant-based, and then the next meal after that, and so on.

Part of change is about setting achievable goals, and if you set the goal of committing to eating plant-based each day, that gives you the opportunity to hit your goals every day and to be constantly building up your conviction. By viewing the change in this more understanding and ultimately achievable way, you are relieving yourself of some of the most daunting psychological aspects of becoming vegan.

In time, once you've adjusted to this new way of living, the prospect of it being a lifelong commitment is far less intimidating and will be something that you're actually enthused by. Taking it one meal at a time also helps with any shame that can arise if you slip up, as rather than thinking, *I've got to start from the beginning again*, or, *I'm such a failure*, you just carry on where you left off at the next meal. In essence, you have the chance to prove to yourself that you can do it the next time you eat, which is a great way of building up confidence and trust in yourself.

All of this involves us being reflective and deliberate, something that most people never are when it comes to their food choices. Most people spend their lives making their food choices on autopilot – they eat what they've always eaten because they've always eaten it. But the process of going vegan means establishing a more conscious approach to what it is that we are consuming. It is this more intentional and purposeful approach that over time helps us change our behaviour and create a new normal.

WHAT ABOUT INCREMENTAL CHANGES?

What if you have more than one relapse and you're worried that you're jeopardising the long-term potential of going vegan? One way of approaching veganism is to make incremental changes over a period of time. For instance, this could include going vegetarian and then going vegan, cutting out different foods one by one, or building up the number of plant-based days per week by starting with one and adding in another day every two weeks.

I was vegetarian before I was vegan, meaning that the change for me was incremental. However, it wasn't a deliberate decision to approach going vegan in this way; it was because I didn't know about the dairy and egg industries and thought that being vegetarian was enough. Once I found out that wasn't true, I then made the change to veganism. If I had learned about the dairy and egg industries at the time I was deciding to go vegetarian, I wouldn't have taken the scenic route to veganism.

The way that you approach going vegan is, of course, up to you; however, I tend to recommend that people try to go fully vegan first, approaching that change with the mindset of one day at a time, then if they find they are struggling, try a different approach. The best option is ultimately the one that you find helps you succeed at being vegan in the long run.

If you find that there is one particular animal product that keeps tripping you up, you could decide to eliminate all animal products except for that one, and then cut that one out in the way that works best for you. Maybe you keep giving in to a cheese craving and then find yourself eating animal products again because your stumbling block is cheese. In this case you could cut out all animal products and then reduce your cheese intake over a period of time. You could pledge only to have cheese every other day, and then once you've adjusted to that, remove it entirely.

If, for whatever reason, you do decide to approach the change to veganism through a more incremental approach, it's important to have clear goals in place and a specific timeframe to work towards. The objective is to become vegan full-time – having this as a clear goal is important throughout the process, as it keeps pushing you to make more changes in order to accomplish it. Without that clear goal, we can become comfortable with the incremental changes we've made and not keep moving forward. If we've reduced our overall animal product consumption, we can start to view that position as a suitable compromise, and we can convince ourselves that because we've done something, that's better than doing nothing, so we maintain our current consumption habits rather than taking the next step in the process to going vegan.

To help with this, as well as having a clear outcome in mind, it's important to have process goals, which are steps along the way to help you get closer to your ultimate goal. For example, your first process goal could be cutting out red meat, your next could be cutting out all meat, and the final one could be cutting out dairy and eggs.

Goals should be specific and measurable. So rather than a process goal being simply to eat fewer animal products, a more effective process goal would be not to eat animal products four days a week. That way it is specific, and you know exactly what is required to meet that goal.

The other important aspect of goal-setting is the timeframe, so that you have a clear and specific understanding of what you are doing and when. So, instead of deciding to go plant-based for four days a week and then 'at some point' go plant-based full-time, set a timeframe in which you go plant-based for four days a week and then after two weeks go fully plant-based.

Having clear timeframes is important because it creates a commitment and it means you can properly prepare in advance. If you know when you are going fully plant-based, that means you can make sure you have all the ingredients and recipes ready, and, as a consequence, you'll have a higher chance of succeeding.

How to speak to friends and family about your decision

In Chapter 5, I go into more detail about the practical aspects of becoming vegan when you are living with or dating non-vegans; however, one of the most crucial aspects of becoming vegan to begin with is communicating that change to the people in your life. When it comes to talking to friends and family about going vegan, it is not uncommon to hope that our enthusiasm and passion for making that change will be reciprocated by the other people in our lives. We might think to ourselves, *When my friends hear about what's happening to animals, they'll change too*. However, while it would be undeniably wonderful if they did show an interest in going vegan too, it's often the case that they don't, which can be disappointing and has the potential to take the wind out of our sails. That's why we have to manage our expectations.

The most important thing is that we focus on what we're doing. In fact, living by example can be one of the most effective and persuasive ways of encouraging other people to reflect on their own actions. Plus, being vegan can give our friends and family an opportunity to try plant-based food for themselves and will naturally lead to some conversations and discussions.

FIRST THINGS FIRST

Before you engage with your friends and family, it's again important for you to be prepared and informed. When you first tell people you're going vegan, it may come as a surprise, and the first thing they might want to know, therefore, is how this change is going to affect their lives and what it means for family meals and socialising. It's important to remember that you going vegan isn't just creating a new normal for you; it's also creating a new normal for the people you are closest to. This is why it's a good idea to have a response to alleviate any worries those people might have.

When it comes to friends and family, make sure to be open and communicate with them that you are making the change – this is especially important if you are going round to someone's house for dinner or if you are eating out. If your friends and family know that you're going vegan, it won't be a surprise when you are next in an environment with them where you are going to be eating. You could always reassure them by telling them that you're happy to cook food for yourself or to bring your own food to any family or social gatherings. This can be especially important for festivities and events like Christmas.

Nowadays, it's so much easier to find plant-based options when you are going out for food. However, if in doubt, just take some time to research what the options in your area are. That way, if you do make plans to get food with your friends, you'll know in advance where you will be able to go. This could be especially important if you tend to go to the same restaurants for food with your family, or if you and your friends always order food from a certain takeaway. If you've already checked to see if the usual spots have vegan options, you can reassure your friends and family that these traditions or social habits don't need to change. If they don't have vegan options, you could always take the time to find alternative venues so that everyone is prepared for any changes.

However, as well as the practical elements, it's important for you to be able to respond to any general health concerns. This is especially pertinent when you talk to parents, caregivers and loved ones, as they may naturally be more concerned that you are going to be healthy and look after yourself. So, even if your motivations for eating plant-based and going vegan are not necessarily because of the personal health benefits, it's still important to know how to make sure you are healthy and getting all the nutrients you need. This is obviously vital if you want to stay vegan and be healthy, but it's also really helpful when it comes to answering any questions from family members. In the next chapter, I go into more detail about this and arm you with the knowledge you need to make sure you are eating healthily.

If your family members do ask you questions about health, it's important to remember that these questions are most likely coming from a caring place. While it may feel frustrating or patronising to be told by your parents that they're worried about you, it's completely understandable that they would want to make sure you are taking care of yourself and are informed about your new lifestyle.

There is a huge amount of misinformation and disinformation about health and nutrition, especially in relation to plant-based diets. When we consider all of the different things that we can read online, as well as the perception that many people have of veganism, it's no wonder that so many people are confused about what a healthy diet looks like and whether or not a plant-based diet can actually be good for you. However, being equipped with the knowledge to respond to questions about protein, calcium, iron, omega-3s and vitamin B12 (see Chapter 3) – the usual suspects when it comes to nutrients and plant-based diets – is a really simple yet effective way of allaying any worries from your family members and encouraging them to be supportive of your decision.

DEALING WITH HOSTILITY

I've met countless vegans who talk about the challenges posed by their family members, with many saying it has been one of the hardest and most frustrating aspects of being vegan. When it comes to family, there's already an established dynamic, and there may well be long-standing frustrations or grievances, so adding veganism into the mix can cause friction and problems to bubble up to the surface.

Because communicating the decision to your family can be so daunting, it can be incredibly disappointing if you tell them you are going vegan and they aren't receptive to you making the change. However, it's important to analyse why this might be the case.

If your family aren't supportive, or are even downright hostile, it's important to try and view it from their perspective. After all, if you're going vegan because of the ethics of what we do to animals and because of the environmental harm caused by animal farming, your parents could interpret what you're saying as an insult about their parenting. One of the primary responsibilities of a parent is to raise their child to be ethically responsible, so if their child then tells them that they've changed their behaviour for ethical reasons, it could be construed that they are essentially saying they were raised to commit unethical and harmful acts. Your decision to go vegan could therefore be interpreted as you believing they are bad parents.

Obviously this is not our intention, and it does not take into account the admitted complexity around the consumption of animal products – after all, eating meat, dairy and eggs is culturally normal, legally allowed and undertaken by the majority of people. When we consider all of the nuance and broader context around animal products, it's clearly not as simple as someone being bad because they're not vegan. However, even though we might not be trying to offend or criticise our parents, rationalising why they might be acting uncharacteristically or in a way that upsets us can make it much easier to understand and deal with.

However, for the sake of protecting these important relationships, as well as to ensure that you stay vegan, it's important to acknowledge why there can be tension and to try and view it from a less emotional perspective. If you find that when you first tell your parents they have questions and worries that you don't know how to answer, that's completely OK. While it's important to be prepared, sometimes conversations don't pan out the way that we initially expected. If something is said that you don't know how to respond to, take some time after the conversation has ended to research the answer. Then, the next time you speak to them about veganism you'll be in a stronger position to answer their questions.

The same is true with friends. Perhaps a friend appears spiteful or is deliberately trying to tease, mock or upset you. This is clearly not acceptable, but if you can try and understand their behaviour, it can make it feel less hurtful. The important thing in a situation such as this is to try and not take it personally and instead remind yourself of the reasons you've made the change. If someone tries to upset you or is hostile towards you, that's a reflection on them, not on you.

Perhaps the friend or family member who is not being supportive is feeling uncomfortable because you being vegan is making them reflect on their own ethics and values. Or perhaps they are acting in an unkind way because they are trying to get you to stop being vegan so things will go back to the way they were previously.

While we might want our family members and friends to go vegan because of all the same important reasons we have, it's also the case that them going vegan too would provide us with an added sense of connection with them. I know from speaking with vegans that they often express how happy it would make them if they could share the experience with their loved ones and how it would bring them closer together. However, it could be the case that our non-vegan friends and family members feel the same way and wish that we would stop being vegan because then a source of disconnection would be removed – things could go back to the way they were and we could feel closer again because we would be sharing the same experiences as we were before.

As well as attempting to rationalise unsupportive or hostile behaviour, there are other ways to help yourself deal with it. First, take a deep breath and a moment to compose yourself. If you don't want to have the conversation with them, try and explain to them that you're not interested in arguing and that you'd appreciate it if they would stop. If you're in the middle of a disagreement and it's going round in circles, you could try and say something along the lines of: 'This is clearly an emotive topic, and it seems that we are talking past each other. I think it would be best if we just leave this conversation for now, and we can always return to it when we are feeling calmer and more relaxed.'

There is also nothing wrong with removing yourself from a situation if the person you are speaking to is being unreasonable. For example, if you're arguing with your parents, you could always step out of the room. If you're with friends, you can remove yourself for a few minutes so that the situation can be de-escalated.

While it is obviously extremely difficult if you decide to go vegan and are then met with unsupportive friends or family members, it could also be the case that over time they soften and become more supportive and accepting. After all, the longer you are vegan, the more and more normal it becomes to the people in your life. This is something that I know many vegans, including myself, have experienced.

HOW TO COMMUNICATE

When it comes to how others react to veganism, sometimes people's responses can arise as a consequence of their expectation of what being a vegan means. While it might be unfair, vegans can suffer from an optics problem, and people often presume that we will be judgemental, self-righteous and preachy. It's not uncommon to hear remarks such as: 'I hope you're not going to become one of *those* vegans.' Or: 'Great, I guess this means that we're never going to hear the end of it now.' These kinds of comments are not particularly helpful or productive, but they do potentially suggest that the person who said them is concerned that the dynamic between you will change. As a consequence, when you tell your friends and family that you are going vegan, it's important that you are mindful of how you communicate this choice to them. You don't want to offend or upset them, nor do you want to come across in a way that fulfils some of the negative stereotypes that vegans can be associated with. In response to a negative remark like the ones above, you could simply say, 'I'm still going to be the same person. I'm going to be making some changes in my own life, but these are not going to change our relationship.'

As well as potentially being on the end of some snarky comments when you first mention that you are going vegan, there's a strong chance that this will be the time when you find yourself facing a selection of questions and anti-vegan excuses. Try to be as prepared as possible to answer some of the more common questions that people might have, but, again, don't worry if someone says something that you don't know how to respond to.

Early on in my veganism, I told some friends about the environmental impacts of animal farming, to which someone replied that I as a vegan was responsible for rainforest deforestation in South America due to my consumption of soya products. I now know that the biggest driver of deforestation is cattle farming, and that the overwhelming majority of soya produced in South America is used as animal feed, but at that point I didn't know how to respond. So, if you are asked a question that you don't know how to answer, that's absolutely fine. In response to such a question, you can say something along the lines of: 'I don't know the answer to that question at the moment. However, when I have the chance, I'll certainly have a look into it and then perhaps we can continue this conversation at a later time.'

Another common response is 'whataboutery', where someone tries to discredit an argument by raising a different issue and attempting to deflect any criticism or difficult questions onto the person they are engaging with, because trying to frame someone as a hypocrite or not perfect is a really simple, albeit disingenuous, way of minimising the credibility of what the person is saying. For example, if you're informing your friends and family that you've gone vegan because of the environmental issues around animal farming, someone might ask you in response if you still drive a car.

If someone engages in whataboutery, you could respond by saying, 'By no means am I saying that there aren't other issues outside of veganism that need to be addressed, and I'm not saying that I'm now perfect because I'm vegan. However, animal exploitation is not only one of the most severe ethical and environmental issues that exists, it's also something I can easily choose not to participate in. I personally believe that just because we can't be perfect doesn't mean we shouldn't try and be better. Don't you agree?'

Another important element to consider when it comes to whataboutery is that it often comes from a place of discomfort. For example, if someone is ethically or environmentally minded and they hear that you are going vegan, this can make them feel uncomfortable about their own actions. Perhaps they feel hypocritical or are experiencing cognitive dissonance as a consequence of your reasons for becoming vegan and eating a plant-based diet. Rather than reflecting on those feelings, the person might then use whataboutery to try and relieve some of their dissonance and reaffirm to themselves that it's OK that they are not vegan.

If you're discussing the fact that you've gone vegan for ethical reasons, you might be asked something along the lines of: 'Do you think I'm a bad person then because I'm not vegan?' A question like this can pose a challenge, as on the one hand you probably don't think they're a bad person, but on the other hand you do think that what we're doing to animals is wrong. With this in mind, you could say something like: 'No, I certainly don't think you're a bad person. I don't think that I was a bad person before I went vegan. However, now that I've become properly informed about veganism and the issues that it addresses, I've realised that it best aligns with my values. If you're at all interested, I would be more than happy to share this information with you.'

By responding in this way, you are taking into account the feelings of the person who has asked you the question without diluting the ethical importance of veganism. You're also stating that the issue is not that people are bad for not being vegan, but that there is a general lack of awareness around veganism itself. Also, by offering to share this information with the person, you are inviting them to learn for themselves without them feeling like they are being forced into something they don't want to engage with.

There is also a selection of general communication techniques that can help you more effectively discuss veganism and the reasons why you are choosing to stop your participation in animal exploitation.

Listen

When you tell your friends and family you're going vegan, make sure to actively listen to what they have to say. This is a really simple yet productive way of signalling your respect to them and allaying any potential concerns they might have. Conversations can become heated and tense when someone fails to listen to what the other person is saying, so avoiding that by not talking over the person you are communicating with and giving them the space to express themselves is important.

Validate

Validating someone isn't the same as agreeing with them or condoning what they are saying – instead it's about acknowledging why they might think or say the things they do. For example, if your parent turns around and says they're worried about you going vegan because of protein, your first reaction might be to get frustrated with them because you know that it's easy to get protein on a plant-based diet. However, reacting this way could make them feel insulted, belittled or *invalidated*. Instead, approach any questions they have with understanding. For example, if they do mention protein, you could reply with: 'I completely understand why you're worried about me getting enough protein. I also used to think that we needed meat for protein. However, you can get more than enough protein from plants – in fact, I would be very happy to talk you through good sources of plant-based protein so that you won't be worried.'

Language

When talking to your friends and family about your change to veganism, being mindful of the language and tone you use is also a simple yet highly effective way of making what you're saying more constructive and appealing. If you approached your friends and said, 'I'm going vegan because everyone who isn't vegan is an animal abuser who should be ashamed of themselves,' that could clearly lead to some rather heated exchanges. However, if you instead said, 'I'm going vegan because I looked into what we do to animals and I realised that ethically it goes against my values. I've always said that I'm against animal cruelty, and because pigs and cows are also sentient beings like dogs and cats, I feel that going vegan is the morally right thing for me to do.'

Body Language

Alongside what we say, the way we communicate non-verbally is also extremely important. Things like shaking your head, appearing irritated, scrolling on your phone, tapping your feet or pointing your finger are all going to contribute to an ineffective conversation. Instead, be mindful of your body language and appear calm by relaxing your shoulders, keeping your hands unclenched, giving eye contact and facing the person you are speaking to. The important thing to remember is it's not just what we say; it's also how we say it and how we present ourselves.

While we might not win over all of our friends and family straight away, by being mindful of how we communicate our decision to them we can at least ensure that we don't inadvertently perpetuate any negative stereotypes. Plus, conversations present us with an opportunity to ease any worries our friends and family might have, and also to educate them about veganism and why we have made the change. While this can certainly be quite daunting, it can be really rewarding and empowering to have productive and meaningful discussions.

WHAT IF I STILL LIVE WITH MY PARENTS?
If you still live with your parents or guardians, there might be some barriers that stop you from being able to make the decision to go completely vegan. Perhaps your family aren't supportive of the decision, or perhaps they are supportive in principle but don't view it as practically possible for them as they don't themselves want to go vegan, and buying in extra food or cooking different meals is not something they are prepared or financially able to do.

However, if you find yourself in that situation, it could be that becoming vegan isn't as inconvenient or practically difficult as it might initially seem. For example, there are often simple ingredient or food swaps that can help make the meals your family eat also suitable for you, such as choosing plant-based butter or margarine over dairy, and vegetable stock over meat-based stock. Also, products such as breads, snacks and condiments are all things that can contain animal products but are also extremely easy to find vegan versions of. So even if your family might not be prepared to get rid of meat, dairy and eggs entirely, there might be a number of very easy swaps that your family could opt for that make no difference to them but would be really helpful for you. And rather than cooking different meals, it could be that they put your portion in a different pan and don't add the non-vegan ingredients. For example, if your family are cooking a stir-fry, they could transfer your portion into a separate pan and then add tofu to yours and meat to theirs.

While this might seem like an extra expense, that's not necessarily the case, because plant protein can actually cost less than animal protein, and if you're simply swapping the protein, your meal could actually end up being less expensive. That being said, if you're after an alternative or something that is more expensive and you have your own source of money, you could offer to buy that product yourself so that you're not costing your parents anything extra. If you know where your family usually get their shopping from, you could also have a look on the website for that supermarket to see how much different foods cost. That way you can tell them how much it will be and if they can save money.

You could also offer to buy products for your family to try themselves, such as plant milks, meat alternatives or plant proteins such as tofu and seitan. That way, you might be able to positively influence them to cook more plant-based meals themselves. You could offer to prepare some meals as well, which gives you the chance to show off how tasty plant-based food can be and is a nice gesture if your family are being generally accommodating to your veganism; for example, by making your food separately.

Your family's concerns might not necessarily be around you wanting to go vegan, but instead because they are worried you expect them to take responsibility for you wanting to change. So if you can also show that you are willing and able to help ease any of the inconvenience or extra considerations that might be involved, then that will only help make you going vegan more palatable to them.

The important thing to remember is that you can only do what you are able to do. If you are unable to go fully vegan because you still live with your parents, then just commit to choosing the plant-based options in all the situations where you can. You can also use that time when you are still at home to become as informed and prepared as you can, so that when you do leave home and become independent, you can then put everything you know into practice and hit the vegan ground running.

Finding your tribe

A really helpful way of making the change to veganism easier is to find like-minded people, as other vegans can be a source of validation, confidence and knowledge.

It can sometimes feel alienating going vegan, even if the people in your life are supportive. You are having to make new decisions, get used to a new way of living and come to terms with the harm that animal exploitation is responsible for – something that you were most likely blissfully unaware of for a long time. All of these things can create a sense of loneliness and isolation.

It can also be hard to break out of a habit if everyone you spend time with is still engaging in it. For example, if you were trying to stop smoking but all of your friends smoked, having all of your social experiences with them would make it extremely challenging for you not to smoke with them too. This would become even more challenging if your friends were tempting you to smoke by asking you to come outside with them or asking if you wanted one. Something similar can happen with non-vegan friends. If we live with or go out to eat with non-vegans, we are constantly surrounded by people engaging in and normalising the behaviour that we are trying to change. They might ask if you want to try some of their food or make comments like: 'Come on, surely you can have just one chicken nugget.' This might not even be said to be intentionally discouraging or invalidating, but it can obviously have that effect.

If you think that your friends or family might try and encourage you to eat an animal product, it's a good idea to have something prepared in advance that you can respond with. For example, you could say something along the lines of: 'Thank you for your offer, but as you know, I'm actually not eating animal products any more, and I would really appreciate it if you didn't offer me any from now on, as veganism is something I feel very passionate about.'

Social pressure, even if it's not overt, has a huge influence on how we think and behave. Being prepared can take away some of those difficulties and give us more confidence if we are in a situation where we are being encouraged to do something that goes against our wishes. Plus, by being polite but assertive we are hopefully asking the people in our lives to be more respectful and not repeat that behaviour again, thus making it easier for us in the future.

Being prepared for social interactions is especially important when we consider that peer pressure can make us do things that go against our better judgement. A study on social conformity found that during a task where a group of people each had to state which one of three lines on a card matched the line on a different card, the participant who was being tested would pick a different and clearly incorrect line if the majority of the other people in the group had done so. When interviewed afterwards, there were participants who said that they had chosen the wrong line even though they were certain it was wrong, simply because they had decided to yield to the position of the majority in the group.

If we can be influenced by other people to choose something that we can see is clearly wrong, it shows how persuasive peer pressure can be in influencing our decision-making. In the case of animal products, this can especially be the case, as the negative consequences of eating animal products are not directly in front of us, which makes it easier for us to rationalise why we are conforming to the pressure being exerted by the group we are in.

This doesn't mean you need to cut yourself off from everyone who isn't interested in going vegan. Instead, it can be helpful to find some like-minded people who you can also chat to or spend time with. That way you can have your decisions validated, rather than constantly feeling like the odd one out. Plus, finding support from other vegans means that you can learn from them too, as they will have experienced many of the same things and will be able to relate to what you're going through. Feelings of isolation are compounded when it also seems like we have nobody in our life who can relate to what we're doing or who we can talk to about it. So one of the primary reasons why finding people on the same wavelength as you is really important is because it provides you with an opportunity to talk to someone who understands and is not going to be confused or judgemental.

As humans, it is important for us to have meaningful interactions with others, which means forming connections based on values and ethics, as well as interests and hobbies. Thankfully, there are lots of vegan groups online, and there are also lots of vegan meet-ups and groups that organise social events where you can hang out with other vegans.

All of this being said, the dynamic of being with non-vegans can also create something positive in relation to behaviour change. When you tell others that you are making a commitment to do a particular thing, you are introducing a very powerful incentive. Once the people in your life know that you are going vegan, you are increasing accountability on yourself and generating a sense of expectation from those in your life.

Reward yourself

This brings me back to a point I made earlier about veganism creating an opportunity for you to feel more confident about what you can achieve. Overcoming any social pressures and difficulties further teaches you about how independent and motivated you can be to do things that are meaningful to you. By sticking to your goals, even when it is challenging, you are constantly showing up for yourself and building trust. You are also proving to the people in your life that you are serious about being vegan and that you are capable of changing your behaviour, despite how difficult this can sometimes be.

In the same way that someone who has pledged to stop smoking will feel immensely proud of themselves if they go out with their smoking friends and don't smoke, the same is true for vegans who have stopped eating animal products. And while your friends and family members might not go vegan themselves, by fulfilling the commitment that you stated you were pursuing, you are also having a positive impact on the way that others perceive you.

This plays into the idea of having a reward incentive. When it comes to behaviour change, having a reward when you meet your goals is a very common tactic to keep you on track. While giving in to some of the initial challenges will lead to a sense of disappointment, the inverse is true when you stick to your commitment.

You can also create a reward system by treating yourself to something every time you hit a milestone; for example, going to the cinema, buying a new video game, visiting a museum or going to a new bar. Combining the behaviour change with rewards gives you clear goals to work towards. You could start by having a reward for when you complete your first week, then your first fortnight, then your first month, and so on.

Embracing the bittersweet

Outside of meeting like-minded vegans, another way to feel validated and to reaffirm why you are going vegan is to meet animals who have been saved from the animal farming industries. Interacting with pigs, cattle, chickens, turkeys, sheep and other animals is an extremely valuable way of connecting with the ethics of veganism. There's a bittersweet undertone to animal sanctuaries, as on the one hand it's really rewarding to be around animals who have been rescued, but on the other hand you are reminded of the animals who have not been so fortunate. This bittersweet feeling is a crucial one to hang on to, and, in many ways, it defines the vegan experience – the sweetness of positive change combined with the bitterness of why that change is necessary in the first place. This duality provides both the imperative to be vegan and the sense of empowerment that comes with it.

Veganism is both an intellectual and an emotional philosophy. The intellectual side solidifies the rational reasons why we need to change, whereas the emotional element encourages us to focus on our feelings and empathy. Going to animal sanctuaries informs both aspects, as we get to meet species of animals that we don't normally encounter, meaning that we can see them act autonomously and showcase their individuality. This adds credibility to the ethics of veganism, while also creating an empathetic point of reference.

If we are in a situation where we are considering eating an animal product, we can think of the animals we met and consider whether we would still be thinking about eating that animal product if we knew it was going to come from them. There are many animal sanctuaries, and a lot of them have open days, tours and volunteering opportunities. Plus, by visiting an animal sanctuary, not only do you get to meet some rescued animals, you can also meet like-minded people at the same time. It's essentially a win-win.

In a nutshell

To summarise, it's important that you approach becoming vegan with understanding and compassion for yourself. Behaviour change can be challenging, and there are a variety of incredibly valid and understandable reasons why this is the case.

To make becoming vegan easier, the first thing to do is become informed about why you are making the change. After that, you want to make sure that you have prepared yourself. This includes: setting realistic and achievable goals that could be tied to a reward system; identifying in advance what might cause you to struggle or what you anticipate you will find difficult; and having strategies and plans in place for if there are any setbacks or mistakes.

Part of being prepared is thinking ahead about telling your friends and family, and trying to anticipate what their reactions might be. Do you think they will have concerns or questions? If so, how will you respond? Will you be able to alleviate any worries they might have, including questions about health and essential nutrients, and more practical questions about eating out and cooking food?

If you think your friends or family might be antagonistic or hostile, can you attempt to rationalise in advance why they might react in this way? If so, can you take that into consideration when you tell them you're going vegan? If you expect that they might try to encourage you to break your veganism or make undermining comments and remarks, do you have something prepared in advance that you could say to them?

It's always important to keep in mind that succeeding at something doesn't mean being perfect or faultless. While you don't want to approach going vegan with the mindset that you will make mistakes, setbacks can ultimately aid in you succeeding because of what they can teach you and how you can use them to your advantage.

Now that we've explored the psychology of behaviour change, as well as some tips and techniques to make becoming vegan easier, let's delve into the practical aspects of going vegan – and where better to start than food?

CHAPTER 3

HOW TO NAVIGATE FOOD

We've discussed the reasons why going vegan is so important, and we've also explored the nature of behaviour change and ways of making the transition to veganism easier and simpler. The next step in this process is to tackle what is the single biggest aspect of going vegan: food.

This is the most important part of the conversation because, in terms of scale and impact, it is the biggest contributor to the problems I've previously outlined. It is also the area of animal exploitation that we engage with the most.

Food is also the most challenging part of veganism, not just because of how often we need to eat, but also because it is the behaviour that is most strongly tied to culture and identity, and therefore the one that elicits the most emotions. It is also the area where there is the most temptation, with advertising, marketing and our own sensory associations with animal-based foods all playing a role in reinforcing the general view that it is OK to consume them because they are tasty and bring us enjoyment.

However, I believe we can flip this around: food is the aspect of veganism with which we can have the most fun and find the most enjoyment too. Trying new flavours, cooking with new ingredients, veganising our old favourite recipes and discovering how life-enriching and enjoyable plant-based living can be are all part of the process of changing our diets. For all of the potential challenges of changing how we eat, there are also the potential rewards and satisfactions that come with changing our food choices.

What do vegans eat?

When we think of vegan food, we probably have a stereotypical image in our head of what it looks like. When I first went vegan, that image was of boring salads, and the stereotype at the time was that vegan food took the fun and flavour out of food and made it dry, bland and unenjoyable. As a consequence, we vegans were very used to hearing jokes about how we ate twigs, grass and cardboard.

On the bright side, at least these jokes signified that some people actually knew what veganism was! In the early days of my veganism, as referenced in the introduction, I lost count of the number of times I asked if there were vegan options in a restaurant or cafe, only to find myself being looked at blankly or being sincerely told that, 'Yes, there are indeed gluten-free options available.' I also had to politely turn down the 'vegan' options that were made from fish on several occasions.

Thankfully, things have moved on, and generally speaking most people have now heard of veganism and know what vegans do and don't eat. The problem nowadays is that vegan food is often tied to processed foods like burgers and other meat alternatives. One of the prevalent worries and criticisms around being a vegan today is the mistaken assumption that being vegan means having to eat more processed food, which is the opposite of the reputation plant-based food used to have.

This is why one of the simplest and most helpful things to start with is to acknowledge that a plant-based diet encompasses a wide spectrum of different foods. Boring salads can be suitable for vegans, as can interesting and flavoursome salads – and plant-based food isn't just salads. Likewise, meat alternatives and products such as dairy-free cheeses are often suitable for vegans, but plant-based food is also so much more diverse than just these alternatives.

One of the most telling things that I hear people say in relation to plant-based food is: 'I could never go vegan because I don't like vegan food.' This means they don't like fruits, vegetables, wholegrains, potatoes, nuts, legumes and the list goes on. In reality, people eat and enjoy food that is suitable for vegans every day. In fact, many meals already consist of a majority of plant-foods, so going vegan is often more about making small tweaks to dishes we already enjoy than wholesale changes. When we reshape what we perceive eating a plant-based diet to be, all of a sudden there's lots of plant-foods for us to enjoy.

This is important to recognise, because veganism is often viewed as changing your lifestyle such that you are going to be eating in an entirely new way when that is not necessarily the case. It also challenges one of the most common arguments against veganism, which is that plant-based food isn't accessible enough, a perception that is again tied to the common assumption that being vegan means eating plant-based alternatives. While most supermarkets do stock these products, it is also true that they are not as generally accessible as the meat, dairy and egg products they are a direct substitute for.

However, if you buy your groceries in a supermarket, then veganism is already very accessible to you, regardless of whether or not the supermarket has a good range of plant-based alternatives. This is because supermarkets also contain a wide variety of different plant-foods.

While it is true that you probably already do eat lots of plant-foods, going vegan does give you the opportunity to try new things and experiment with ingredients in a way that you might not have before. This is a really fun and enjoyable part of becoming vegan – you might find a new food that you had never tried before but end up really liking. For me, there were a number of foods that I never ate before going vegan, such as tofu, tempeh, lentils and even lots of different vegetables and fruits. Early on after going vegan, I realised that when I'd eaten animal products, I was just eating the same foods that I had always eaten, with very little variation or experimentation.

People often argue that going vegan means restricting your food options, and while this is technically true, in the same way that it is technically true that laws prohibiting us from eating dogs, cats, dolphins and whales restrict our food options, many vegans find that they actually start eating a wider range of foods and ingredients than they did before. If you think about the animal products that people mainly consume, they tend to eat a fairly narrow range of species, especially when viewed against the enormous number of different animals we could technically eat but don't consider to be food. However, by removing these animal products and finding foods to replace them with, all of a sudden there are a far greater number of choices. We could choose a plant-based alternative that is directly meant to replicate the animal product we're no longer eating, or we could choose a plant protein such as tofu, tempeh or seitan, or legumes such as beans or lentils, or a combination of different plant proteins.

By removing the animal product, we are creating space on the plate for something else, and the options for what it can be replaced with are potentially far more varied than we might have initially realised. This brings me back to the section in Chapter 1 about the health benefits of eating plant-based, in which I outlined how removing animal-based foods is a win-win from a health perspective, as it means removing products that have been linked to increased chronic disease risk and replacing them with a healthier alternative.

WHAT IF I DON'T LIKE A PLANT-BASED PRODUCT?

Through this process of experimentation and trying new ingredients and foods, you might try something and realise that you don't like it. In fact, there's a very strong likelihood that you won't like every alternative or plant-food that you try, and that's completely fine. However, the chances are that there were some meats or cheeses you preferred to others, or even animal products that you simply didn't like. When I was younger, I enjoyed eating doner kebabs, but I didn't like the flavour of a lamb's leg or a lamb steak.

It's important to approach plant-based food with the same mindset. You might cook a recipe or try a product and just not enjoy it. However, sometimes with new ingredients it's about learning how to cook them. The first time I tried tofu I did not like it, but then again I just opened the packet and cut a portion off and ate it on its own. Plain tofu straight out of the packet is not the best way to eat tofu! Once I started marinating, seasoning and cooking it, I realised that tofu is actually incredibly versatile and very enjoyable too.

There's a wide range of flavours and textures within the plant kingdom, some that you will prefer over others. The same is true with plant-based alternatives as well, and there are also differences in terms of overall quality in the alternatives sector, meaning that some products are just generally better than others.

The important thing to remember is that you might try a vegan cheese you don't like (believe me, we've all been there), but that doesn't mean that you won't like all vegan cheeses. Similarly, you might buy a plant-based meat alternative and think it's not very good, but that doesn't mean that all meat alternatives are the same. And it could also be the case that you try an ingredient like a type of bean or vegetable and you don't particularly like it – that's absolutely fine too.

When I first went vegan, one of the foods I wanted to have a plant-based version of was a cheeseburger. So I began my pilgrimage to my local health food store – vegan options were far less available than they are now, which meant that health food stores were usually where you could find vegan chocolates, cheeses and meats. Once there, I found a packet of plant-based burger patties and some vegan cheese. *This is going to be easy,* I thought to myself as I paid for the products.

I then proceeded to stroll nonchalantly home, shaking my head from side to side in a playful public expression of my disbelief at all the needless fuss and hubbub that is made about going vegan. *People just need to chill out – this vegan thing is a piece of egg-free cake,* I thought as I opened my front door and proceeded to the kitchen to turn on the hob and get the frying pan ready.

The first tickle of doubt emerged when I opened the packet of vegan cheese and gave it a smell. *The smell and flavour probably develop once it's had a chance to breathe. A bit like red wine,* I thought, as I quickly moved on to frying the burgers. The smell did not improve. I knew the game was up when I attempted to slice the cheese, the chalky and crumbly texture revealing that there was more chance that Piers Morgan would go vegan than there was that this vegan cheese would melt.

Rather than taking a nibble of the cheese then and there to try it, I gamely decided that there was nothing else for it:

I'd make the cheeseburger as I'd intended and take a big bite out of it without spoiling my palate beforehand. Perhaps the cheese didn't smell, look or feel good, but nestled in a bun, with some ketchup, lettuce and a plant-based patty, it would defy the odds and surpass my now extremely low expectations.

I plated the cheeseburger up, sat down and took a bite. *Oh no,* I thought.

In the beginning, going vegan can be a process of trial and error. There will be some new foods that you really like, some you're ambivalent towards and some you don't like at all. Over time you'll find your favourites and get to know which ones aren't your cup of tea. Speaking of which, don't be disheartened if the first plant-based milk you make a cup of tea with curdles. This used to be a common problem for vegan tea drinkers, but nowadays it's easy to get plant-based milk that doesn't curdle. You can even get plant milks specifically designed for cups of tea.

The quality of plant-based alternatives is improving all the time. So, even though there might not be a good and readily accessible vegan alternative for every animal product that you can buy, things are getting better and will only continue to do so. This means that some of the flavours and textures that you might initially miss are not necessarily gone for ever. Getting a delicious plant-based cheeseburger is incredibly easy now. So don't lose hope if you sit down to eat a vegan version of one of your favourite meals and rather than feeling satisfied, you are left facing an existential crisis.

Another thing to bear in mind is that if you go from eating animal products straight to plant-based alternatives, you will most likely be hyper-aware of any differences between the two. Yes, plant-based alternatives are improving in quality all the time, but that doesn't mean that every single one is going to feel and taste exactly the same as the product it is replicating.

Sometimes it can be valuable to think of plant-based alternatives not in terms of whether they taste identical to their meat counterparts, but whether they taste good on their own terms. I have found that this can be really valuable in the case of vegan cheese. Truth be told, at the time of writing, vegan cheese still has some work to do. However, it is much better than it was ten years ago, and it is going to continue getting better. There are many types of vegan cheeses now available that are tasty in their own right. They might not always replicate the salty and fatty tastes or textures that we commonly associate with cheese, but that doesn't mean that they are not enjoyable to eat.

I find it helpful to think of the animal-based product that the alternative is replicating as more of a guide as to how the alternative can be used. For example, if a plant-based product is marketed as being like beef, whether it be a burger, mince or steak, this can be used as an indicator of how it can be used as an ingredient and what type of recipes it would be a good addition to. Some of the most enjoyable meals I've had with alternatives have been enjoyable, not because the alternative was exactly like a piece of meat I used to eat, but because the alternative was just genuinely delicious. Plant-based milks are a great example of this, as different plant-based milks have different flavours and are tasty in their own right, not because they taste like cows' milk.

So having a point of reference is helpful because it informs us consumers what these alternatives are suitable for and the types of meals they are intended to be included in. However, one of the drawbacks with this is that it can create an expectation that the product isn't able to live up to. While we don't necessarily have the expectation that milk made from soya should taste like cows' milk, our expectation of a chicken or beef substitute made from soya tends to be slightly different.

This is not to say that there aren't some genuinely convincing plant-based alternatives on the market, and having products that provide the same flavour and texture as animal-based foods is important if you once enjoyed those types of foods. However, the plant-based food sector also provides the opportunity to widen the number of foods and flavours available to us. For example, in the same way that there are a wide variety of different types of meat-based sausages available, plant-based sausages can be viewed as an extension of this variety, except they are made from plants and not animals. Some of these sausages will taste the same as the meat-based ones and some will have their own flavour.

In essence, trying new foods can lead to both disappointment and enjoyment. There'll be some new foods that you will find tasty, and some that you might not like as much. The important thing is not to be disheartened if you try a new food and don't enjoy it. Instead, you can always try different alternatives and ingredients until you find the ones that you do like.

BUT ISN'T PLANT-BASED FOOD MORE EXPENSIVE?

One of the most common arguments against plant-based diets is that they will end up costing you more. But is this true?

The simple answer is that it depends. There are undeniably expensive plant-based foods on the market, particularly some artisanal nut-based cheeses and certain plant-based alternatives. Some alternatives can be more expensive than animal-based foods due to a smaller supply chain, supermarket margins and other economic factors. However, these are not foods that you need to eat regularly, if at all, in order to be a vegan.

A vegan diet is also sometimes considered to be expensive because of people's perceptions about what it entails. Plant-based diets have commonly been linked to wellness and celebrity dieting, which brings with it the association of privilege and being out of touch.

However, just as before, the best way to challenge the myth that plant-based diets are inherently more expensive is to survey exactly what foods can be included in a plant-based diet. By doing this, not only can we begin to make plant-based eating seem more accessible, we can also begin to recognise how cost-effective eating plant-based can be. After all, beans, lentils, wholegrains, starches, vegetables and fruits – the core food groups in a healthy plant-based diet – are often among the cheapest foods that you can buy.

A 2021 study from the University of Oxford showed that pescatarian diets were the most expensive and wholefood plant-based diets were actually the most affordable.[1] In fact, in high-income nations, a wholefood plant-based diet was shown to reduce food costs by up to one-third when compared to a standard omnivorous diet. So, even though there are some plant-based products that are more expensive, because you can actually save money by eating plant-based, you may well be able to treat yourself to some artisanal nut-based cheeses from time to time precisely because you are saving money elsewhere.

When I hear this argument, I am often reminded of a joke that I heard growing up: 'Why don't we eat venison? It's a little bit dear.' Tastelessness aside, it does reinforce the wider point I'm making – there is a spectrum of costs associated with animal products as well as plant products, and in the same way that it would be unrepresentative to claim that eating meat is always expensive because of the price of deer flesh, it is also unfair when veganism gets labelled as expensive because of the price of certain plant products.

READING LABELS

When you first go vegan, it can be a little daunting knowing what packaged foods you can and can't eat. For example, while many breads are vegan, you're still going to want to check because not all bread is. Thankfully, packaging has improved a lot over the years, which means that many foods now have clear labels that state whether or not the product is suitable for vegans. Most supermarkets also now have their own vegan ranges and sometimes even dedicated vegan or meat-free sections, meaning the vegan products can usually be quite easy to spot.

That being said, vegan products are often put with vegetarian and gluten-free products, so even if something is in a vegan section, it can still be a good idea to double-check before buying it. This is especially the case if the section is labelled as meat-free rather than vegan. Also, it's becoming more common for supermarkets to place vegan products in the aisles where the animal-sourced products are. For example, plant-based mince is sometimes placed alongside the animal equivalent. While this can be more inconvenient for us vegans, from a marketing perspective there is evidence that it can increase the number of sales of the plant-based product.[2]

Not long into my veganism, I made the mistake of presuming that a packet of falafel was going to be plant-based. Just before I was about to dip the first piece into a tub of hummus, a thought crossed my mind to check it was vegan after all – both milk and eggs were listed as ingredients. Since then, whenever I've thought about just picking something up and presuming it is vegan rather than checking that it definitely is, I remind myself of falafel-gate.

Milk powder is one ingredient to definitely keep an eye on. In fact, it's a rite of passage for new vegans to pick up a product that they presume is going to be vegan, only to then find that for some reason beyond comprehension milk powder is listed as an ingredient.

As well as checking labels in order to double-check something is definitely plant-based, I would also recommend checking labels on items that you presume are not going to be suitable for you to eat, as sometimes foods you might not expect are in fact vegan. This can include foods that are meant to have a cheesy or a meaty taste, or foods that you would presume would contain dairy or eggs, like certain biscuits. It can be quite surprising what foods are suitable for vegans by chance rather than design, and because these foods were not created for vegans, they often don't carry a vegan label or any type of certification on them. Also, sometimes foods that are suitable for vegans are only labelled as vegetarian, so it can be worth checking these products out too, just to see if they are suitable or not.

The good news is that the more labels you check and the more used to it you become, the easier it gets as you become a more proficient label reader. This means that although it can be a little inconvenient at the beginning, it doesn't stay that way for long. While in most cases you would only need to check the label once to know if it is suitable, it can be a good idea to double-check products from time to time, as companies can sometimes change their ingredients. This is particularly relevant in products that are vegan by default rather than design, as companies are less likely to be thinking about these products from the perspective of making sure they are suitable for vegans.

Because of allergy laws in the EU (which were retained in the UK after Brexit), the 14 major food allergens are bolded on ingredients labels. This can also be very helpful for us vegans, as it means crustaceans (such as prawns, crabs and lobsters), eggs, fish, milk and molluscs (such as mussels and oysters) should by law appear in bold on ingredients labels so that they stand out and are easy to spot. If you see any of those animal products in bold, that tells you straight away that the food isn't vegan, but if none of these animal products are listed, the next step is to have a read through the rest of ingredients to make sure that there are no other animal products included.

The highlighting of food allergens might not always be the case when you are travelling, though, and it doesn't necessarily mean that these animal-product allergens will be listed on menus in restaurants, takeaways and cafes. The good news is that most places that have vegan options will highlight those options in some way. However, if you're ever in any doubt, there's no harm in asking a server or staff member just to confirm that something is vegan. For example, if I'm ordering a coffee with milk, I'll often just double-check that the staff member heard my order correctly by saying something along the lines of, 'Sorry, just to double-check, that was with oat milk?' Or, if the coffee has already been made and is being handed to me, I might say, 'Is that the oat-milk coffee?'

Here's a list of other terms and words to be mindful of:

Dairy-free and Lactose-free
These terms don't necessarily mean that a product is vegan. In the case of lactose-free, the product might even be dairy-based still.

Whey, Lactose and Casein
These are all ingredients that come from dairy.

Albumen
Another word for egg white.

Vitamin D3
There are two types of vitamin D: D2 and D3. D2 is vegan and is the type of vitamin D that is used to fortify foods that are suitable for vegans. You can also get vegan versions of vitamin D3, but most vitamin D3 that is added to food is produced from lanolin, which comes from sheep's wool. It is easy to get a vegan vitamin D3 supplement to take yourself, but most foods that are fortified with vitamin D3 use an animal-derived version. To make things a little more complicated, often these fortified foods just say vitamin D and don't clarify which type. However, unless the product states that it is suitable for vegans, it is more than likely that the product is using animal-derived vitamin D3. Vitamin D3 from lanolin is suitable for vegetarians, making it even more important that you check a product is also suitable for vegans.

Lanolin
As just mentioned, lanolin is sourced from the wool of sheep. However, not only is it used to produce vitamin D3, it can also be found as an ingredient in cosmetics. This is because lanolin is a grease that is secreted by animals that produce wool and so is sometimes used in moisturisers and other cosmetics because of its wax properties.

Honey, Beeswax, Bee Pollen, Royal Jelly and Propolis
These are all ingredients derived from bees.

Gelatine
A thickening agent made from the skin, bones and connective tissue of cows and pigs. It is commonly used in sweets.

Shellac and E904

Shellac can be used as a glazing agent in foods such as confectionery, chocolate and chewing gum. It can also be used in cosmetic products, including lip gloss and nail varnish. It is derived from a resin that is secreted by the female lac beetle. Even though the beetles don't technically have to be killed for the resin to be acquired, the harvesting process results in the deaths of many of the animals. Interestingly, the Vegetarian Society of the UK used to allow their Vegetarian Society Approved trademark to be used on products that contain shellac, but at the start of 2022 they changed their policy and no longer certify goods that contain the ingredient.

Carmine, Cochineal and E120

These are all different names for the same ingredient, a red dye that is created from cochineal insects that have been ground up to create a dark red powder. It is used as a food colouring and also in some cosmetics.

WHAT ABOUT 'MAY CONTAIN'?

One of the most common and understandable questions that people have when they first go vegan and start reading labels is: 'What does "may contain" mean?' And if something 'may contain' an animal product, does that mean it is not suitable for vegans?

The 'may contain' part of a label can be confusing at first. However, just because something 'may contain' milk or eggs, for example, does not mean that the product isn't vegan. This is because the 'may contain' phrase is a precautionary allergen warning and is there to warn consumers that there has been the potential for cross-contamination. This is normally due to the manufacturing process, whereby a product could in theory come into contact with an allergen that isn't one of its ingredients. This can apply to plant-based foods, as they are often made in factories that also use animal products. So, while the food itself is suitable for vegans, there is still a chance that cross-contamination could have occurred. However, the risk is low, and purchasing the products in question doesn't mean supporting animal farming. Unless you have allergies to the ingredients listed in the 'may contain' section, there's no reason for you not to buy the product.

A more grey-area situation arises when ordering plant-based foods that are cooked on the same grill or fried in the same fryers as non-vegan foods. For example, when Burger King in the UK launched a plant-based Whopper, the burger was labelled as not being suitable for vegans because, even though the patty was plant-based, it was cooked on the same grill as the meat-based patties.

This is similar to 'may contain', as even though animal products aren't part of the food, there could be cross-contamination. However, if vegans can eat 'may contain' foods from supermarkets, you might be asking yourself why they can't eat 'may contain' foods from takeaways. This is why it's a grey area, because eating a product that could be cross-contaminated is not causing more animal exploitation, suffering or slaughter, and it's not contributing to any of the environmental problems related to animal farming either. Yet many vegans wouldn't order something if they knew it was cooked in this way, because they'd be too worried about eating an animal product.

If something is cross-contaminated in a factory, it's probably not going to be noticeable and you're probably not going to be able to taste it. However, accidentally eating a small piece of meat or dairy cheese is most likely going to be far more obvious. So, from a personal perspective, it makes sense why vegans would draw a distinction. However, from a more objective point of view, because the concept of 'may contain' means that you're not actually driving the demand for animal products, eating a plant-based product is still technically vegan, even if it's cooked on the same grill, in the same way that it's still vegan even if it was produced on the same production line as something non-vegan.

Ultimately, the most important thing is choosing the plant-based option. If you're out with some non-vegan friends, or hungry and struggling to find any plant-based food, there's no reason why you should place an extra strain on yourself.

The Burger King example was a really clear case of potential cross-contamination, to the extent that they made a point of telling people about it, so there was naturally more awareness around the possibility of it being an issue. However, when you go to a restaurant and order a plant-based meal, because you don't tend to know how the food is being prepared, you might feel less conscious of cross-contamination, even if that doesn't necessarily mean there is any less of a chance that it has occurred.

Personally, if I was forewarned that the vegan food I was ordering was cooked using the same equipment as animal products, I would be worried about accidentally eating a piece of an animal or the food taking on those flavours. However, I've also eaten at restaurants or ordered food from takeaways and had no idea whether or not the food was cooked using the same cooking equipment, and as a result have not given it a second thought.

We don't live in a vegan world, and we can't always eat food from vegan-only places or establishments that make sure to prepare the plant-based food separately. So, even though we might ideally want to avoid cross-contamination, it's not always easy to do. Plus, because cross-contamination means that you're still not actively participating in the animal farming industries, it comes down to personal choice at the end of the day.

An interesting offshoot from this particular conversation is the wider question of whether or not vegans should be eating from places like Burger King in the first place. This sort of question often comes up within the vegan community, as it presents an ethical dilemma. On the one hand, these companies are among the worst offenders when it comes to their exploitation of animals, yet on the other hand, we want plant-based food to be more accessible so that it's easier for people to choose a plant-based option.

When I was a teenager, I used to go to McDonald's regularly with my friends. If I had wanted to go vegan back then, one of the biggest obstacles would have been the social aspect. At a school talk I gave in early 2025, one of the students asked me if there were vegan options in fast-food chains, and the question caused me to reflect on when I was this student's age and would go to McDonald's with my friends.

It may be seen as hypocritical for vegans to eat at these places, considering that all their business models are built on the very thing that vegans seek to oppose. However, this way of thinking also creates a slippery slope – after all, when we go to supermarkets to buy plants we are also supporting companies that engage in animal exploitation.

Some vegans argue that we should prioritise vegan businesses wherever possible, but this isn't necessarily doable, and if you're the only vegan in your friendship group or family, only ever eating in vegan restaurants is going to be extremely challenging. Plus, if we want to encourage more people to eat plant-based options, that means having plant-based options available in places that non-vegans eat at and enjoy. If those options aren't supported or there is no demand, companies won't provide them, making veganism less accessible overall.

This is another one of those grey areas that has credible arguments on both sides. If you want to avoid these companies, there are of course strong and justifiable reasons that underpin that feeling. However, if you're someone who used to eat at Burger King or McDonald's, then you don't need to stop because you've gone vegan.

WHAT IF THERE IS FOOD LEFT OVER OR GOING TO GO TO WASTE?

Another interesting question that new vegans often have or find themselves faced with is: what about food that is left over and going to waste? Is it ethical for a vegan to eat that food even if the food has animal products in it?

When you have first gone vegan is the time when you might find the prospect of eating animal products the most appealing, but doing so runs the risk of jeopardising your abstinence from animal products. In the previous chapter, I discussed that challenging our perception of animal products can be a really effective way of ensuring you go and stay vegan. So if we consume animal products, even if we have not contributed to the supply, we are still viewing animal products as a food that we want to eat. Think of it like this: if there was dog or whale meat on the table, would you still choose to eat it to avoid it going to waste?

While choosing to eat animal products in this situation might differ from giving in to a craving and ordering and consuming something animal-based specifically for yourself, it still presents a risk when it comes to relapsing on your veganism in general. There's also the message it sends out to those around you. I referenced previously that when I first went vegan, I visited a friend's house and spoke about how much I wished I could have some of the steak they were cooking, and how doing so reinforced to my friend that being vegan was unpleasant and unappealing. If we happily and willingly choose to eat animal products in front of our friends and family, we are suggesting through our actions that we want to eat these foods and that being vegan is a form of deprivation.

On the flip side, if you turn down the offer of animal products, even if you have not contributed to the demand for animal farming, you are again showcasing your commitment and desire to stay vegan. In other words, it sends out a strong message. This is especially important, as sometimes people can use situations like this to test the edges of your commitment by trying to get you to renege on your decision.

At the end of the day, if someone orders too much food and can't finish it, that's their waste, not yours. It's also highly likely that the person whose waste it is could simply leave it and finish the food off later when they are hungry again.

WHAT ABOUT ALCOHOL?

While alcohol is vegan, not all alcoholic drinks are. This is because certain ingredients and agents can be used in the production of some alcoholic products. Those that can be ruled out easily enough are the ones that contain milk, cream and honey. One of the most obvious examples of this is Bailey's, which contains dairy, although they do also have a vegan option. A less well-known example is low-alcohol beers. This is because alcohol adds body to beer, meaning that low-alcohol beers can become thin and lack the conventional mouthfeel of alcoholic beer. To get around this, some companies add lactose to their low-alcohol beers in order to add more weight and make them more similar to their alcoholic counterparts. There are a number of low-alcohol options that are suitable for vegans, but it is advisable to check beforehand.

Some cocktails contain egg whites, again to change their texture. Due to egg being an allergen, it is standard practice for cocktail bars to list egg as an ingredient. However, if you're unsure, you can always just ask the bartender or server to confirm that there are no egg whites included.

A vegan alternative to egg whites in cocktails is aquafaba, which is the water that legumes have been cooked in. However, you don't actually need to cook the legumes yourself to get aquafaba, as you can get it straight from tinned legumes. Aquafaba from tinned chickpeas is one of the most commonly used forms, as it has a neutral taste and look. Aquafaba can also be used as an alternative to eggs in baking and cooking, meaning it can be used to make vegan meringues and cakes. Plus, because it is essentially a waste product, it's also an extremely cost-efficient substitute for egg whites. Alongside making a delicious homemade hummus, you can also save the chickpea water from the tin and make a smooth textured cocktail to go alongside it and some meringues for a sweet treat.

Beers and wines can be slightly more confusing. At their core, they are vegan, but sometimes animal-derived ingredients are added in the latter stages to clarify the drink and to create a clear and consistent finish. The most common of these ingredients is isinglass, which is derived from the swim bladders of fish. Alcohol isn't as clearly labelled as food products, meaning that it is not always the case that ingredients like isinglass are listed. However, it is extremely easy to get beer and wine that is suitable for vegans, and it is common now for brands to advertise that their products are suitable for vegans on either the packaging or online. So if you have a favourite brand of beer, wine, ale or stout, just have a look on the brand's website to see if they state that their products don't use isinglass or other animal-derived ingredients. And because isinglass comes from fish who have been killed, if alcoholic drinks are labelled as vegetarian, there is a good chance that the drink is suitable for vegans too.

There is also a really useful website called Barnivore (www.barnivore.com) that has a database filled with tens of thousands of alcoholic drinks and tells you whether or not they are suitable for vegans.

What should I expect when I go vegan?

Often when the health benefits of veganism are discussed, people talk about how going vegan made them sleep better, boosted their energy and improved their skin. While all of these things are entirely possible and do happen to some people when they go vegan, I think it's always wise to approach plant-based diets with the perspective that these things might not happen to you. I hope they do, but it's not a given, and if you go into veganism with the expectation that you will feel noticeably different, you're potentially putting too much pressure on yourself. If you're then left feeling disappointed, that's hardly a positive emotion to carry with you into your veganism, especially during times where you suffer any setbacks or are struggling with cravings and motivation.

Too often when we hear about diet and lifestyle changes we are bombarded by other people sharing their experiences. In the same way that I could tell you stories about how eating plants made me feel better, you could also find people saying that a carnivorous diet or drinking urine did the same for them. Anecdotes are compelling because they're personal and relatable, and they're also easier to understand than complex nutrition science. However, they can also be dangerous because people can end up believing things that are simply not true, allowing bad actors to influence people in ways that are harmful. So, while going vegan can bring about noticeable health benefits in a short period of time, anecdotes are among the weakest form of scientific evidence, which is still true even when those anecdotes support our own position.

The reason I bring this up is because I have been asked on a number of occasions to describe the noticeable changes that I felt when I went vegan. I try to answer this question by bringing it around to the wider and more important part of this conversation, which is what the body of evidence shows us about the healthfulness of plant-based diets: first, that we can be healthy vegans, and second, that taking out animal products from our diets can also reduce our risk of developing many of our most common chronic diseases and killers. The important thing to remember is that those two things remain true even if we don't necessarily feel any different.

To answer the wider question of what to expect when you first go vegan, because you are eating more fibre and potentially consuming more water too, especially if you are eating more fruits and vegetables, it might be the case that you see a change in your bowel movements. However, this is nothing to worry about. Generally speaking, people don't consume enough fibre, even though it is incredibly important for a wide variety of reasons, including improving gut health and reducing the risk of chronic disease.

How to eat healthily

One of the most common and also important questions around becoming vegan is how to eat healthily. While it is true that plant-based diets can improve our overall health and wellbeing, it is also true, as it is with any type of diet, that you can become deficient in essential nutrients if you don't ensure you are eating in a healthy and nutritionally balanced way.

So, how do you make sure that you are eating healthily on a plant-based diet?

CALORIES

When you go vegan, one of the first things to be mindful of is making sure that you are eating enough. This may seem like an obvious thing to say; however, plant-foods generally have fewer calories than animal-derived foods. This means that if you are going from eating cheese and red meat to eating more beans and pulses, your diet might end up having fewer calories in it.

If your GP has suggested you lose some weight, then this can be really helpful, as you can eat until you are full but be consuming fewer calories than you were previously. If you don't want to lose weight, though, then this is something to be mindful of.

When I first went vegan, I went from eating lots of creamy sauces, chocolate, fried eggs and halloumi and other cheeses to making meals consisting of ingredients such as quinoa, kale and beans. Cheeseburger disaster aside, I used my shift to veganism as a reason to eat healthier too. But while these new meals had the right foundations, many of the new meals and foods that I was consuming had fewer calories than the ones I had been consuming previously. This meant that I ended up constantly hungry and not feeling satiated after I had eaten.

This can be a common response from people who have just gone vegan. They find it difficult to feel full and don't stay feeling full for as long as they used to. To make it easier to eat enough calories, incorporate some high-calorie plant-foods, such as nuts and nut butters, dried fruit and seeds into your diet. Wholegrain foods are also really helpful in this regard, as not only are they healthier than refined carbohydrates, they also contain more nutrients and higher amounts of protein and fibre, both of which can help you feel fuller for longer. So swapping grains such as white rice for brown rice and white pasta for brown pasta is not only a better option from a general health perspective, it will help with making sure you feel satiated too.

It's also worth noting that our bodies adjust over time. When you first change what you're eating, especially if you weren't eating many wholegrains, legumes and vegetables before, you might notice a difference in regard to how full you feel, but over time your body adapts. The important thing is to ensure that you are eating your recommended daily intake of calories. If you're unsure, you could always track your calories for a short period after making the transition to make sure you are getting the amount you need.

NUTRIENTS

One of the positive things about the health scrutiny around plant-based diets is that you can use it as encouragement to learn more about how to be healthy. Before I was vegan, I knew very little about different nutrients and what a healthy diet looked like. However, the desire to go vegan coupled with the fact that plant-based diets are often thought of as lacking in essential nutrients meant that I ended up learning things I wouldn't have otherwise.

One of the most frustrating phrases used by advocates of animal products is that eating meat, dairy and eggs means you are eating a 'balanced diet', implying that a plant-based diet is unbalanced and, as a result, unhealthy. However, this is an outrageously oversimplified way of viewing diet and also misrepresents nutrition science, which shows you absolutely can be healthy and plant-based. It's also dangerous, as it creates the impression that simply by eating animal products, you'll get all the nutrients you need, when this isn't necessarily the case. The truth is that you can eat any type of diet and be deficient in key nutrients. There are anaemic meat eaters and there are anaemic vegans. There are vitamin D-deficient meat eaters and vitamin D-deficient vegans. There are vitamin B12-deficient meat eaters and vitamin B12-deficient vegans. The list goes on.

One way to simplify replacing nutrients is to make like-for-like swaps. So, if you are replacing meat in a meal, rather than replacing the meat with a vegetable, replace it with a good source of plant protein instead. Here are some key nutrients to be mindful of and good plant-based sources.

Protein

When you go vegan, one question that you will almost certainly be asked is: 'Where are you going to get your protein from?' This question persists because there is such a strong association between animal products and protein, and so there is, sadly, a false belief that getting protein from plants is difficult. Thankfully, this is not the case. There is actually protein in all plant-foods, although the amount can vary, meaning that it's advisable to incorporate some plant-foods that are particularly good sources of protein into your daily diet.

Sources of plant protein include:

- Soya products such as tofu, tempeh, soya milk and soya yoghurt
- Legumes such as beans, lentils, chickpeas and peanuts
- Seitan (a protein source made from wheat gluten)
- Wholegrains such as quinoa, buckwheat, brown rice and wholewheat pasta
- Plant-based alternatives such as burgers, sausages, mince and 'chicken' pieces

Sometimes people worry that plant proteins are not complete proteins, meaning that they don't contain enough of all the essential amino acids our bodies need. However, there are actually plant-foods that are complete proteins, such as quinoa, soya products and buckwheat. That being said, even though you can get complete plant proteins, this isn't necessarily relevant, as you don't need to get all the essential amino acids from just one food item. The important thing is that you can get all the essential amino acids you need from a plant-based diet by eating a variety of plant-foods in a day and by making sure you are eating enough calories for you individually.

Calcium
We tend to associate dairy products with calcium; however, you can get calcium from plant-based sources, including:

- Fortified plant milks and dairy alternatives
- Legumes such as white beans, chickpeas and soya beans
- Vegetables such as broccoli, kale and spinach
- Nuts and seeds such as almonds, sesame seeds and tahini
- Fruit such as figs, oranges, blackberries and blackcurrants

The easiest way to get enough calcium is simply to consume a fortified plant-based milk in the situations where you once consumed cows' milk, because plant milks are fortified in such a way as to ensure that they are providing comparable levels of calcium to dairy. So, by consuming these dairy alternatives, alongside other calcium-containing foods such as those I just listed, you'll be ensuring that you have enough calcium in your diet to be healthy.

Vitamin D
This vitamin is related to calcium, as it helps optimise its absorption. The main source of vitamin D is direct sunlight, as our bodies can produce vitamin D when our skin is exposed to the sun. The good news is that it is estimated that just 10 to 30 minutes of sun exposure between 11am and 3pm is enough for most people in the UK, for example, to produce the vitamin D they need.[3][4] This is just as well, as too much sun exposure can be harmful, so protecting yourself from the sun is also important when it comes to skin health and cancer risk.

In many parts of the world, sunlight can be inconsistent, especially during the colder and darker months. Dietary sources of vitamin D are also not especially abundant; oily fish and eggs are the foods most commonly associated with it. However, as mentioned previously in this chapter, you can also get vitamin D from fortified foods. As vegans, we just have to be mindful of whether or not this vitamin D is animal-derived. The easiest way around this is to opt for fortified foods that are labelled as vegan, such as plant-based alternatives like plant milks and yoghurts.

The most effective way of getting enough vitamin D is to take a supplement, which is recommended whether you're vegan or not. This is because it ensures you are getting a consistent and standardised dose every day. Even during the summer it can be helpful, as you might work inside or not be able to get direct sunlight during the peak hours. I'll talk more about supplements in a moment, but opting for one with a vegan source of vitamin D3 is the best option.

Iron

Iron is an incredibly important part of our diets, especially for menstruating women. In fact, while women who no longer menstruate and men need around 8.7mg a day, women who menstruate need 14.8mg a day.[5] Among other things, our bodies use iron to make haemoglobin in red blood cells, which carry oxygen in our blood.

There are two types of iron: haem and non-haem. Haem iron comes from animal products and non-haem iron predominantly comes from plants. Even though we generally associate dietary iron with red meat, it is possible to get all the iron that is needed through a plant-based diet, which is especially important considering the evidence that links red meat with chronic disease.

Fortunately, iron can be found across a wide spectrum of different plant-foods, including:

- Plant proteins such as beans, lentils and tofu
- Vegetables such as kale, garden peas and spinach
- Nuts and seeds such as cashews, pumpkin seeds, hemp seeds and flaxseeds
- Fruits such as dried apricots, dried figs, tinned tomatoes and black olives
- Wholegrains such as oats, quinoa and spelt
- Fortified foods such as bread, cereal and wholewheat biscuits
- Other sources of iron include dark chocolate, blackstrap molasses and dried thyme

Vitamin C can also increase iron absorption, and if there's one nutrient that plant-based diets are never accused of lacking, it's vitamin C. This is because vitamin C is abundant in fruits and vegetables, meaning that something as simple as adding broccoli or bell peppers to a dish, squeezing lemon juice over a meal or adding some berries to your breakfast can help increase the amount of iron that is absorbed.

Omega-3
There are three main omega-3 fatty acids: ALA, EPA and DHA. ALA, which is a short-chain omega-3 fatty acid, is found mainly in plant-foods, especially flaxseeds, chia seeds, hemp seeds and walnuts. The body can convert ALA into the long-chain omega-3 fatty acids EPA and DHA; however, the rates of conversion can vary.

The reason we normally associate omega-3 with fish and fish oil is because they can provide us with preformed EPA and DHA. However, fish do not produce these fatty acids themselves – these nutrients instead originate from algae. So when we get EPA and DHA from fish, we are essentially filtering the nutrients through fish unnecessarily. In the same way that it is extremely common for people to take fish oil supplements, vegans can instead take an algae oil supplement to get preformed EPA and DHA, which is a great way of complementing the EPA and DHA that is converted from the ALA we get from plants.

SUPPLEMENTS

The fact that vegans are recommended to take supplements sometimes leads to the criticism that a plant-based diet can't be healthy. However, vegan or not, we all rely on supplements and fortified foods to some degree, whether it be a vitamin D supplement that is advised for everyone, or the fortification of soils and food that occurs throughout the supply chain in order to boost nutritional intake and make it easier for consumers to get the essential nutrients they need. So a vegan taking a supplement or eating a fortified food is no different to a meat eater taking a supplement or eating foods that are fortified. Also, the animals we farm are given supplements, drenches and fortified feed, so even the nutrients people get from animal products can be the result of fortification and supplementation.

The simplest and most practical way to tackle supplements is to take one specifically formulated for vegans. While it is possible for vegans to get all the nutrients they need if they are consuming fortified foods, a supplement that covers the nutrients that vegans should be most aware of is a simple way of helping to make sure that you are hitting all your nutrient goals. As a general rule, a good targeted supplement for vegans would contain vitamin B12, vitamin D3, DHA and EPA, iodine and selenium.

One of the biggest issues around nutrition and diet is how intricate and precise it can be. We can become hyper-fixated on ratios and nutritional profiles, and it can become quite overwhelming and tiring. Before I went vegan, I spent very little time thinking about nutrition, and the truth is, I don't spend much time thinking about it now. However, as a result of going vegan, I am far more informed than I used to be, and the fact that I don't spend much time overanalysing my diet is more to do with feeling confident than it is about me being dismissive.

So, while it can feel a little intimidating at the beginning – and you might be hearing about nutrients you've never heard of or thought of before – once you are in the groove of eating plant-based and feel confident you are getting the nutrients you need, including taking any supplements, it feels much easier.

There are also apps that allow you to track the food that you eat and will measure the nutrients that you are consuming so that you can see if you're hitting your needs for the day. And if you want to make sure that you are not low on any essential nutrients, you could always get a blood test once you've been vegan for an extended period. That way, you can make any adjustments if you need to. It's also reassuring to know that health authorities including the NHS and the British Dietetic Association support the position that a plant-based diet can be healthy.

It's also important to bear in mind that health is bigger than just diet alone, so reducing stress, exercising regularly, socialising and taking time to do things you enjoy are all a part of living a healthy life too.

Also, if you want to, it's absolutely fine to indulge in some vegan ice cream, cookies, doughnuts, burgers and sausages from time to time. While a healthy plant-based diet is one that focuses primarily on whole plant-foods, that doesn't mean you need to avoid unhealthy foods altogether. We all deserve a treat now and again.

BUT WAIT, SHOULDN'T I BE AVOIDING ULTRA-PROCESSED ALTERNATIVES?

There is a lot of merit to the concern about ultra-processed foods (UPFs), which can be low in essential nutrients and fibre, and high in calories, salt and sugar, making them extremely unhealthy. There's no denying that foods including biscuits, doughnuts, cakes, sweets and microwaveable meals made with processed meat and refined carbohydrates are not good for us.

However, there is vagueness about what constitutes ultra-processed, and grouping a whole range of very different foods under one classification is reductive. The problem is not simply that foods are processed, but instead what that processing means in terms of the ingredients, nutritional profiles and subsequent health outcomes associated with those foods. Creating a binary distinction between unprocessed and processed can ultimately lead to conclusions that are actually more harmful overall.

One clear example of this is plant-based alternatives and meat. For example, a review study of the research that has been carried out on plant-based alternatives, meat and heart health found that plant-based alternatives were associated with better overall cardiovascular health than meat products, including unprocessed meat.[6]

We also see this problem play out within individual food categories as well. Categorising all foods within a food group as being equally bad from a health perspective just because they're ultra-processed completely ignores the differences between items. Grouping all plant-based alternatives together overlooks the fact that there are also huge differences between the many varieties available. Some are healthier than others; for example, some contain less salt, some contain higher amounts of fibre and some are fortified with essential nutrients like iron and B12.

Today, one of the primary food categories people most associate with UPFs is meat alternatives. Many of these alternatives are replicating animal-based UPFs such as bacon and sausages. Yet, while health guidelines focus on the need to reduce these animal-based foods, media reporting often centres around plant-based alternatives being the types of UPFs that consumers should be most concerned about.

Sadly, this narrative is creating a huge amount of confusion among consumers and has become a sensationalist talking point, as demonstrated by how a 2024 study looking at UPFs was covered in the media. The researchers found that increased consumption of plant-sourced UPFs led to an increase in the risk of cardiovascular disease and death. However, the plant-sourced UPF category included vodka, fizzy drinks, cakes and biscuits, and these foods were not necessarily even vegan, as they just had to be of 'primarily plant origin'. This means that chocolate biscuits containing milk could have been included in the plant-sourced category.

Plant-based meat alternatives were also included in the plant-sourced UPFs; however, they only accounted for 0.2 per cent of the calories consumed by those being studied. To make matters worse, the meat alternatives in the study also included tofu and tempeh, which are not normally considered to be ultra-processed and are considered healthy plant proteins. In reference to plant-based alternatives, the lead author of the study also stated that they couldn't 'draw specific conclusions related to this particular type of food'.[7] However, this didn't stop headlines such as VEGAN FAKE MEATS ARE LINKED TO INCREASE IN HEART DEATHS[8] and VEGANS ARE SLOWLY KILLING THEMSELVES.[9]

There is also a false impression that unprocessed foods are always going to be healthier than processed foods, but this isn't the case. Red meat may be unprocessed, but that doesn't mean that it is healthy – it has still been shown to increase the risk of cancer[10], heart disease, hypertension, type 2 diabetes and more. However, due to the ultra-processed conversation, many people now have the impression that processed meat alternatives are unhealthier and worse for your body than unprocessed red meat.

Somewhat ironically, when plant-based alternatives were less healthy than they are now, the public perception of them was far more favourable, mainly because the media reporting and general conversation around them was more positive. These foods were seen as an exciting form of food technology and a disrupter that offered significant potential when it came to addressing the ethical, environmental and health issues associated with animal products.

That narrative has now shifted for the worse, even though many plant-based alternatives have gotten healthier. For instance, Beyond Meat have reduced the saturated fat content of their burgers by 60 per cent and salt by 20 per cent. Their latest burger even has endorsements from the American Diabetes Association and the American Heart Association.[11] All of this just shows how important the messaging around foods really is, as the issue is not necessarily the products themselves, but the perception the public has of them.

Alternatives can also be good sources of essential nutrients. They tend to have comparable levels of protein to their animal product counterparts, and they usually contain or are fortified with other nutrients that you might normally associate with animal products. For example, meat alternatives can contain iron and vitamin B12, and plant milks are often fortified with calcium, as well as B vitamins and vitamin D. This can be really helpful, as it makes it easier to replace those nutrients. In the case of plant milks especially, as mentioned earlier, because dairy is a source of calcium, using a plant milk that is fortified with calcium makes it really simple to ensure that you are still getting enough calcium in your diet (see also the list of calcium sources earlier in this chapter).

Gellan gum is added to some plant milks, as it allows the calcium to be distributed equally throughout the product. However, plant milks are often labelled as being ultra-processed because of this ingredient, further emphasising the danger of deciding the healthfulness of a product based on whether it can be technically labelled as ultra-processed or not. Calcium is an essential nutrient, and gellan gum is considered a safe food additive. A study showed that even when people ate close to 30 times more gellan gum per day than typically found in a normal diet, there still weren't any negative health outcomes.[12]

You can get plant milks that contain fewer ingredients and are not ultra-processed, but those plant milks will often not be fortified, and as a consequence you are missing out on an opportunity to have an easy source of calcium, vitamin D and certain B vitamins. However, from a health perspective, opting for the no-sugar versions of plant milks is advisable.

The reason all of this is important is twofold: first, because it's important to challenge the misinformation that exists, and second, because these alternatives can be helpful if you are missing the taste and texture of animal products. While whole plant-foods are still the healthiest options, and opting for legumes, nuts, wholegrains, fruits and vegetables is preferable, incorporating some alternatives into your diet is also absolutely fine. As mentioned earlier, not all alternatives are the same. So, if you are looking for healthier alternatives, you can always opt for those with lower salt and saturated fat content, as well as higher fibre and added fortification.

That being said, if you're not interested in eating meat and cheese alternatives, that's also absolutely fine – with the exception of fortified plant milks, which are recommended, other alternatives are by no means a requirement for a plant-based diet.

What about cell-cultured meat?

Cell-cultured meat is created from the cells of actual animals and is real animal meat. However, it doesn't come from a slaughtered animal, as the process of producing it does not require an animal once the cells have been acquired. So, is cell-cultured meat vegan?

If veganism from a food perspective is defined as simply not eating anything that comes from an animal, then cell-cultured meat is not vegan. However, this overlooks a crucial question: what is the real purpose of going vegan? The philosophy of veganism is about opposing the exploitation of animals, which currently means avoiding the purchase and consumption of animal products.

There's a very clear reason why meat isn't vegan – it requires the exploitation and slaughter of animals. But what if it didn't? The issue with meat is not the meat itself, but all of the things that are required for that meat to end up on our plate. However, if you remove the animal exploitation and slaughter, you potentially remove the ethical issues around eating meat. This is why the question of whether cell-cultured meat is technically vegan overlooks the more important question of whether or not it is ethical.

One of the main ethical drawbacks with cell-cultured meat has been the use of foetal bovine serum, which is even worse than it sounds – it is taken from the hearts of bovine foetuses during the slaughter of pregnant cows and is used as a growth medium; however, there are now plant-based alternatives that are being used instead. This removes the most significant ethical concern around cell-cultured meat.

In reality, the biggest obstacles facing cell-cultured meat are not its ethical merits, but the funding that is still required to get it to market, and the political and social pushback that is attempting to frame it as something to be avoided. Cell-cultured meat isn't being produced for vegans – it's primarily being made for people who aren't vegan, which means its success rests on it becoming accepted by society at large.

Personally, I think cell-cultured meat is a symbol of some of humanity's best traits and some of its worst. I say worst because I think it is a real shame that we 'need' to develop cell-cultured meat to stop the exploitation of animals. This is indicative of the self-centred and myopic behaviour patterns that our species are often plagued by. However, cell-cultured meat is also an intellectual marvel. The fact that we are able to create such a product speaks to our ingenuity and ability to problem-solve and find solutions for the betterment of our species, and indeed other species too.

Cell-cultured meat is often labelled as unnatural, but modern-day farming and food in general are all products of technology and scientific understanding. Farming by its very nature is unnatural, as it is a product of our manipulation of what is natural. This is by no means an inherently bad thing, as what is natural is very rarely what is preferable. Case in point, we have medicines to treat natural diseases, we live in homes with heating and electricity, and we have sanitation systems and consistent access to clean drinking water. If what is natural is what is preferable, not only would we be arguing against all of the life-improving examples I just listed, but we would be forced to reject many more as well.

While cell-cultured meat is plagued by insinuations of it being an unearthly creation made by ethically ambiguous scientists in laboratories, the actual process of creating it is not quite so science fiction as it might sound. The animal cells are grown in tanks known as bioreactors, which are similar to those used in breweries to make beer; however, rather than alcohol being fermented, it's meat instead.

As things currently stand, this is more of an interesting thought experiment than it is a tangible choice in front of us. However, that might change in the future. Cell-cultured meat has been granted regulatory approval in several countries around the world, and in the UK cell-cultured pet food went on sale for the first time in early 2025.

If cell-cultured meat can overcome the obstacles it faces, it stands a real chance of becoming a significant disrupter to our current system of food production. Whether or not to eat it would then become a matter of personal choice for each vegan. You might decide that you want to try it, or you might not see the value of it and give it a miss. One thing is for sure, though: if we reach a point where cell-cultured meat is commercially viable and socially accepted, its potential to reduce animal exploitation is absolutely massive.

What should I cook?

Throughout this chapter, I have gone through all of the main considerations relating to veganism and food. However, there is still one overarching point to cover: what does all of this mean when it comes to the actual meals you will be eating?

In the previous chapter, I discussed the importance of preparation. Part of this was thinking ahead about what meals you could cook and buying ingredients in advance so that you minimise any potential issues that you might encounter. What these plant-based meals are is entirely up to you and will depend on your time, budget and what foods you like.

One really simple way to find vegan recipes is to look online, as it is a fast, free and easy way of seeing what recipes suit your needs and sound appealing to you. There are websites dedicated to plant-based recipes, such as BOSH! (www.bosh.tv) and Deliciously Ella (www.deliciouslyella.com), and many major recipe websites have a great selection of plant-based recipes too, such as BBC Good Food (www.bbcgoodfood.com). If you have a few meals that you used to really enjoy – for example, chicken korma or spaghetti bolognese – search online for vegan versions of those. In fact, one of my favourite meals before I went vegan was spaghetti bolognese with garlic bread. The good news is that it still is one of my favourite meals now that I am vegan because I can just eat a plant-based version instead. So, when thinking about what recipes to find and meals to cook, just think about what meals you already like and find a plant-based version to make instead. Going vegan isn't about reinventing the wheel, and although it's really fun to experiment and try new flavours and ingredients, you can also stick to what you know and already like.

The same also applies to cakes, pastries and desserts. If you have a sweet tooth, find vegan recipes for the desserts and sweet foods that you love. I mentioned aquafaba earlier in the chapter, and there are vegan replacements and swaps that you can use for all the animal-derived ingredients commonly used for baking and desserts. So, fear not if you are a lover of panna cotta, cheesecake, Eton mess or chocolate fudge brownie – you can eat even the most decadent, creamy and rich foods as a vegan.

To simplify things and get you started, in the Resources section of this book there is a meal plan template that you can use. I've also included a list of suggestions for dishes that you could make below, which includes many of the meals that I personally love to cook for myself. One simple tip to make these meals different and more varied is to experiment with the ingredients – that way you are trying different flavours and making it easier to cover all your nutrient bases. An example of this is the recommendation to eat 30 different types of plants a week. So, rather than always cooking with the same ingredients, try and incorporate a range of different proteins, herbs, spices, vegetables and so on.

If time is a concern, you can prepare something that will last multiple days. This can be really helpful with lunches, as you can make them in advance and then you don't have to worry about what you're going to have every day. If you want to add some variation, you could incorporate different additional ingredients each day. For example, if you were making a stir-fry to last several days, you could add crushed peanuts and chilli one day, cashews and spring onions the next day, and sesame seeds and coriander the day after that.

BREAKFAST

- **Porridge** with plant-based milk, berries, flaxseed (which is high in fibre and the omega-3 fatty acid ALA) and nut butter, of which there are now a number of varieties, and which are delicious and filling. I personally love the traditional peanut butter (although peanuts are technically legumes, not nuts), but you can also try almond, hazelnut, cashew and more. There are also seed butters, including hemp and pumpkin seed. This is a really healthy way to start your day and is a great meal when it comes to mixing it up and finding different variations. You could change what plant milk you use; you could use different berries and fruit; you could opt for hemp seeds rather than flaxseed; or, as previously mentioned, you could use almond butter instead of peanut butter. You can also make overnight oats, which is essentially a no-cook way of making porridge. Instead of cooking oats, you soak them in a plant milk overnight and the oats absorb the milk and soften. Similar to cooked porridge, you can add fruit, nut butter, flaxseed, plant-based yoghurt or whatever extras you like.

- **Chia seed pudding,** which you make by combining chia seeds with a plant milk and leaving it in the fridge overnight, just as you do with overnight oats. You can also add some maple syrup if you want it a little sweeter. Not only is this a really quick and simple breakfast to prepare, it's also healthy and easy to customise. Similar to porridge, you can add different types of fruit and nut or seed butter.

- **Scrambled tofu on sourdough bread.** Scrambled tofu is a high-protein, healthy and tasty alternative to scrambled eggs. It can also be used in a similar way by having it on toast or as a side to a larger savoury breakfast, such as a vegan full English. It's super easy to make, as you just crumble tofu into a frying pan with some oil to lightly brown it, pour in some plant milk that has been mixed together with some spices, such as turmeric and paprika, and then fry it until the scramble reaches the texture that you like. If you want to take it to the next level, you can also add some tahini to the plant milk and spices mix, as this makes it creamier, and you can use kala namak (often referred to as black salt), which creates an eggy aroma and taste due to its high sulphur content.

- **Cereal with plant milk.** It might not be that exciting, but sometimes you need something quick, easy and convenient. To make it healthier, opt for wholegrain cereals that are low in sugar. You could also add some fruit on top and some flaxseed or hemp seed. Watch out for the added vitamin D that I discussed earlier, as it can be a sign that the cereal isn't suitable for vegans.

LUNCH

Sandwiches and wraps. If you're not sure what to do for lunches, then why not just keep it traditional and have a tasty plant-based sandwich. You could make it with vegan cheese and meat alternatives, or if you want something more wholefoods, you could make it with tofu or crushed chickpeas with vegetables. Tofu is a very versatile ingredient, meaning that you can use and flavour it in a number of different ways. For example, you can marinate it with your preferred flavours, such as a spicy mix, sweet and sour, Asian-inspired, barbecue, etc. You can then fry it in a pan or bake it in the oven and make it crispy. For chickpea sandwiches, you can simply mash cooked chickpeas with a fork or potato masher and season with the herbs and spices you like the most; for instance, you can opt for something more Mediterranean and season with oregano and add some fresh tomatoes and olive oil, or you can combine the chickpeas with celery, red onion, dill, a squeeze of lemon and a dollop of vegan mayonnaise. If you want your fillings wrapped up rather than between two slices of bread, mix it up and opt for a wrap or burrito instead. You could make a burrito with beans, quinoa and bell peppers, or a wrap with falafel and hummus. Sandwiches, wraps, burritos, flatbreads, pita and any other bread-based food options offer a simple potential for lunches but with lots of room for variation and experimentation.

- **Buddha bowls.** When it comes to healthy, fresh and delicious plant-based lunches, you can't go wrong with a buddha bowl – a typically meat-free meal made up of ingredients that focus on healthfulness and variety served in a bowl. Plus, the sky is the limit when it comes to what ingredients and flavours you can use. A good way of approaching a buddha bowl is to split it into different elements so that you are incorporating a range of foods. For example, a wholegrain, such as brown rice or quinoa; a protein, such as tofu, tempeh, chickpeas, black beans or seitan; vegetables, such as carrots, broccoli, sweetcorn or kale; and healthy fats, such as avocado, hemp seeds or nuts. These healthy fats can also be viewed as toppings, so you could add some chopped walnuts, ground flaxseeds or flaked almonds on top of the bowl. You can also get creative with the sauce or dressing you want to use, opting for a vinaigrette, satay sauce, soy sauce, a spicy dressing or a vegan Caesar dressing, to name but a few.

- **Salads.** If you're looking for something simple that can be made fresh or in advance, salads are a great option. Salads can have an unfair reputation for being boring or for not being filling; however, this doesn't have to be the case – they can be packed full of flavour and also make for a very satisfying lunch. They're also easy to load up with vegetables, wholegrains, pulses, nuts, seeds and herbs. If you're looking for inspiration, you can make plant-based versions of traditionally non-vegan salads such as a Caesar, Waldorf or niçoise, or you can experiment and create one using your favourite ingredients and salad dressings. You can also make pasta salads and add vegetables, vegan cheese and tofu, seitan or a meat alternative to get some added protein. Also, using

wholewheat pasta is a super simple way of adding more protein, fibre and nutrients to your diet.
- **Soups.** Making nutritious and tasty plant-based soups is incredibly easy, and there is so much potential for variation when it comes to all the vegetables and ingredients you can opt for. To increase the amount of protein, you can add tofu, beans or lentils. You could also add a slice of bread for dipping, or garnish with some croutons.

DINNER
- **Pasta.** From the previously mentioned spaghetti bolognese to carbonara and lasagna, you can have a vegan version of all your favourite pasta recipes. For mince you could use a plant-based meat alternative, crumbled tofu or lentils. You can also use soya mince, which is often sold as either textured vegetable protein or dehydrated soya, both of which sound completely unappealing and do not do justice to the food in question. Dehydrated soya is extremely high in protein and is great in meals where you need a mince alternative.

If you want a creamy pasta sauce, you could use soya cream, or you can soak cashews and then blend them with a plant milk. There are lots of different vegan cheese options you can use, including mozzarella and parmesan, and a product called nutritional yeast, which again doesn't have the most appetising name, but tastes cheesy and is great to use with pasta dishes. As mentioned previously, opting for brown and wholewheat pastas is a great way to make the meal healthier. Alternatively, you can also get pasta made from different plants like lentils and chickpeas. These are great if you want to add more protein to your diet; however, the texture can be different to wholewheat pasta. If you want something even quicker and easier, then you can always pick up a pasta sauce from the supermarket, as there are many vegan-by-default pasta sauces. Leftover pasta is also a great lunch option.

- **Curries.** There are so many flavoursome and delicious curries that can be made plant-based, or even come plant-based as standard. If you need a cream alternative, using coconut cream or a different plant-based cream is a really simple and easy swap. Instead of meat, you could add a meat alternative or use tofu. Alternatively, you could add in legumes like chickpeas or lentils.
Curries are also great when it comes to adding lots of vegetables, herbs and spices. Plus, rather than using white rice as a base, you could use brown rice or a different wholegrain like quinoa, which is also higher in protein. Just like with pasta sauces, there are a number of plant-based curry sauces that you can buy from the supermarket.

- **Stir-fries.** Making a stir-fry vegan is exceptionally easy. There are lots of stir-fry sauces that you can buy in supermarkets that are plant-based, and there's also a huge variety that you can make yourself as well. Substituting the meat for a plant protein such as legumes, tofu, tempeh or a meat alternative is an easy way to veganise a stir-fry. You can also swap out white noodles for a healthier alternative such as buckwheat or wholewheat noodles. You could also use a wholegrain like quinoa or brown rice.

- **Stews and casseroles.** Plant-foods are perfect when it comes to creating hearty, rich and flavoursome stews and casseroles. These types of dishes are not only simple, but there are so many different options. You can make chunky potato, celery and carrot casseroles, cooked in vegetable stock with lentils, onion, chopped tomatoes, bay leaves and rosemary. You can do something similar but with plant-based sausages and make a sausage casserole, or you can make Ethiopian-inspired stews using lentils, French-inspired cassoulets or bourguignons, Moroccan-inspired chickpea tagines or plant-based chillis, shepherd's pies and ratatouilles.

- **Burgers and hot dogs.** Maybe you fancy a treat, maybe you have some friends coming over or maybe you're going to a barbecue – thankfully, there are many ways that you can make delicious plant-based burgers and hot dogs. You could experiment with different toppings and fillings, and you can also make some delicious accompaniments such as a plant-based coleslaw or potato salad.

All of this is just scratching the surface of what is possible when it comes to plant-based meal options. For example, as well as looking up recipes and buying ingredients in advance (see the Resources section for some ideas of where to find good online recipes and places to buy vegan ingredients), there are also recipe boxes that you can have delivered with vegan meal kits. These can be extremely convenient, as they provide you with all the ingredients and the exact quantities you need, and they come with recipe cards included. You can also order plant-based food using delivery apps, so if you'd rather just order food in one evening, then that's entirely possible too.

Whether you want to get creative and make completely new meals, veganise the meals you already like, take advantage of deliverable recipes kits or do a mixture of all these options, with a takeaway or two thrown in there for good measure, there is no shortage of ways to eat a delicious and varied plant-based diet.

What about eating out?

So when it comes to eating food at home, there are many options available. The good news is that it has become so much easier to find vegan options when you are out and about as well. This can obviously depend on where you live and what restaurants you have nearby; however, most chains in the UK now have vegan options and sometimes even entire vegan menus, and independent restaurants and eateries very often have options for vegans too. You might even be surprised where you can find good vegan options. I've had some amazing plant-based meals in restaurants and pubs in rural areas where my initial assumption was that I was going to struggle to find something that I could eat.

There is a website and mobile app called Happy Cow (www.happycow.net) that is designed specifically to help you find vegan restaurants and cafes. I use Happy Cow regularly, as do many vegans I know, as it is incredibly useful and makes finding places to eat really simple and convenient.

Even if places don't have clearly labelled vegan options, it could be the case that they can make something suitable for you if you ask. Similarly, if a meal in a restaurant is being planned in advance by friends, family or work colleagues and you don't have a choice about where it is taking place, you can reduce the risk of not being able to eat anything by checking beforehand to see if the restaurant has any vegan options. If they don't, but you get in touch with them in advance and give them some time to prepare, they might be able to make something especially for you.

As with cooking food at home, a little bit of research and preparation goes a long way. So take a few minutes to see if your favourite place has vegan options, or what there is in your local area. If you're out and about and looking for somewhere to eat, a quick search online is also a really convenient way of finding something vegan.

Travelling

Depending on where you are visiting, travelling as a vegan can sometimes be more challenging, especially if the place you are going to is not as vegan-friendly, has fewer vegan options or doesn't have the same labelling laws and guidelines. This can be especially true if you don't understand the language.

However, there are some simple and easy ways to make travelling less challenging and more enjoyable as a vegan. The first thing is to do some research in advance – are there any vegan restaurants where you are going or restaurants that have vegan options? It can make things significantly easier if you have an idea of where you are going to eat and have a plan in place beforehand. You don't necessarily need to plan meticulously everywhere that you are going to go, but if you know what areas have more options and what vegan brands to look for in supermarkets and shops, it can make things less stressful when you are away.

There are now vegan travel apps available, such as the previously mentioned Happy Cow, that show you where vegan restaurants are and also non-vegan restaurants that have vegan options. These can be great if you're planning in advance, and can also be really helpful if you find yourself feeling peckish while you're out exploring on holiday. You can also find translator apps that are really helpful, and which are especially useful for scanning labels in supermarkets.

Another tip is to find out what traditional dishes from the place you are visiting are either already plant-based or can be easily made plant-based. This means that if you find yourself in a situation where there are no vegan restaurants and no vegan options labelled on the menu, you might already have an idea of what is vegan by default or what can be made vegan with relative ease. For example, when I visited Puglia, a southern region of Italy, finding a delicious plant-based lunch was especially easy, as one of the most famous regional dishes in the area is focaccia barese – a traditional dish of focaccia bread, tomatoes and olives. Not only is it plant-based by default, it's widely available in the region, inexpensive and absolutely delicious.

While veganism might sometimes seem like a modern term or concept, eating plant-based food is something that has been commonplace in many countries and cultures for a long time. This means there are many different dishes from around the world that are already suitable for vegans. There's also no harm in asking. If you find a restaurant you like the look of, you can always ask if they have vegan options or can make anything vegan for you.

Travelling can actually provide a good opportunity to try even more plant-based food. There are many places in the world that have a varied and abundant selection of plant-based restaurants and options, especially if you are visiting major cities such as Berlin, Amsterdam, London and New York. So, rather than travelling always meaning that you will find it more difficult to eat plant-based, it can sometimes be the case that going on holiday can make eating plant-based even easier than you have been used to.

Hopefully you are now feeling prepared and equipped when it comes to the food side of being vegan. Like I mentioned at the start of this chapter, what we eat is the biggest element of veganism, and the one that comes with the most challenges. However, there is so much that can be fun and life-enriching about eating plant-based too. A survey of Veganuary participants revealed that 70 per cent of those who took part reported feeling more inspired in the kitchen. And out of the participants who remained vegan after the month of January, the number one thing that influenced their decision to continue was that being vegan was easier than they'd expected.[13]

Approaching plant-based eating can be a little daunting at first, but rest assured that it's actually easier than many people perceive that it will be. So, put aside a bit of time to find some new recipes, ways to veganise some of your old favourites and what vegan options are available where you live. And most of all: have fun, don't be afraid to experiment, and remember that every meal is a chance to positively influence the world around you.

CHAPTER 4

BEYOND FOOD

One of the most important reasons I wanted to establish the difference between a plant-based diet and veganism in Chapter 1 is so that we don't overlook all of the issues that exist beyond food. It might have the most significant impact when it comes to animal exploitation; however, food is a symptom of a wider problem – that we view non-human animals as having such little worth that we have consequently found a wide range of different ways that we can use them for our own personal gain. If we were to view other animals as possessing moral worth that elevated them beyond the status of property or objects, the idea of forcing them into gas chambers would be obviously and clearly unacceptable to us.

It is the denigration and devaluing of animals' lives that has allowed us to create these mammoth industries of mass and systematic exploitation, of which food is the biggest culprit. However, having this mindset towards animals has led to other significant cases of exploitation too, and because veganism is about trying to tackle the fundamental problem and not just addressing some of the symptoms, it encompasses these other areas as well.

Thankfully, it is far easier to make changes in our lives that help us avoid the consumption of non-food animal products. There's a good chance that you might already be engaging in some of these practices, as it has become increasingly common for people to opt for cruelty-free cosmetics and to avoid going to places like aquariums that keep dolphins and whales, even if they are not yet vegan themselves.

Clothing

Outside of food, clothing is the next largest area of animal exploitation that veganism addresses. The ubiquitous nature of animal-derived clothing is in many cases tied to the farming of animals for food. This means that shifting away from animal farming for food will naturally lead to a shift away from many forms of animal-derived clothing. That being said, some animals are raised and exploited purely for their feathers, skins and fur, so the problem can't be addressed by eradicating animal farming for food only. Even when the farming of animals is being carried out primarily for their flesh, the extra income provided from the sale of the animals' hides or other body parts all contributes to the continuation and perpetuation of animal exploitation more generally. All of this means that changing how we buy clothes is another aspect of becoming vegan, as it is a core tenet of living in a way that minimises animal exploitation.

There are a wide of variety of companies that make clothing, footwear and bags that are suitable for vegans, including almost all high-street stores – although there are vegan boutiques that are ethical from a human-labour perspective as well. You can also find items made from non-animal-derived materials in thrift stores. Even brands that use leather or other animal-derived fabrics will often have products that are vegan-friendly. So if there is a brand you like, or if you are looking for a particular item, then searching online is a really easy way of finding a suitable version of what you want and discovering which brands offer products that are suitable for vegans. Searching online can also be extremely useful, as it allows you to be even more specific when it comes to what you're looking for. For example, you can search for organic or recycled materials.

With this in mind, here are the main animal-based fabrics to avoid and what should you look to purchase instead.

FUR

Animals killed for their fur include mink, foxes, rabbits, raccoon dogs, coyotes and more. Of all animal-derived forms of clothing, fur is the one most generally viewed as being unethical – and for good reason. Fur farming is incredibly cruel, with it being standard practice for animals to be confined in tiny cages. They are usually killed by having their necks broken, by being anally electrocuted or by being forced into gas chambers. Fur farming has been banned in the UK since 2000, although it is still legal for fur to be imported and sold there.

Alternatively, furs are taken from animals who have been hunted by trappers who use devices such as leg-hold traps. Trapped animals not only suffer because of the pain of the traps, they also experience psychological distress, which can lead to them damaging their jaws trying to pry the traps open or even biting off their own limbs, which might free them but then ultimately leads to a slow and painful death.

While fur is generally now sold as a designer item in the UK, with a hefty price tag and an underlying sense of entitlement attached to it, real fur can sometimes be sold without people realising what they're buying. Investigations in the UK have found real fur being mis-sold as fake fur at some of the biggest and most well-known clothing brands and street markets. The items in question tended to be smaller and lower priced, such as fur trims on hats and gloves, pom-poms on hats and clothing, and fur trims on footwear. Part of the confusion came from the expectation that real fur is always expensive, which is what the retailers argued in their defence, as they also claimed to be unaware that the products they were acquiring were actually real fur. However, in reality, real fur can often be produced more cheaply than fake fur because of how appalling the farming of the animals is.

Sometimes these products are not mislabelled but simply don't say whether they are real fur or not, meaning that many consumers will just presume that the fur is not real, even though it might be. This is because non-compliance with labelling laws has been shown to be widespread in the UK, with little being done by local authorities to ensure enforcement.[1]

All that being said, the number of times that investigations have shown that real animal fur is being mis-sold as fake fur are few in comparison to the amount of fake fur being sold generally. While this is certainly reassuring, there are also a few simple techniques you can use to find out if a product is real or not. For example, you can look at the base of the fur. If the fur is attached to a mesh or thread fabric backing, it's most likely going to be fake. If it is attached to something that looks like leather/skin, then it is probably real. You can also check out the tips of the hairs – real animal hairs taper to a fine point whereas faux fur typically has blunt ends that don't change in diameter.

In its own defence, the fur industry often says that it is 'natural' and 'eco-friendly', positioning itself as being better than faux-fur alternatives. The claim that it is natural is both irrelevant when it comes to its sustainability credentials and also disingenuous. Fur is natural on animals, but once it is torn off their bodies it will rot unless it goes through a chemical treatment process, which can include the use of formaldehyde and chromium. Plus, a cradle-to-grave study that analysed mink-fur and fake-fur products from their production all the way to post-consumer final disposal found that the environmental impact of real fur is at least three times higher than the least-sustainable faux-fur variant. For some specific environmental impacts, the impact of real fur is more than ten times greater.[2]

Although faux fur is conventionally made from synthetic materials such as polyester, the issues related to those fabrics do not justify the production and wearing of real fur. However, if you are looking to purchase a fake-fur item, you could always opt for something made from cotton or recycled polyester in order to reduce the environmental impact further. There are also innovative forms of faux fur being developed, including fabrics made from plants such as hemp seed and flaxseed. And attempts to produce cell-cultured real fur are also currently underway.

LEATHER

While fur is the animal-derived fabric that people most commonly agree is unethical and is not therefore worn as frequently as it once was, leather is far more ubiquitous, being most often used in footwear, belts, jackets and bags. The majority of the world's leather comes from cattle, meaning that the ethical and sustainability issues surrounding beef are applicable in the case of leather as well. However, some people try to make a distinction between beef and leather, meaning that it is not uncommon for even vegetarians still to wear leather products.

This distinction is based on the false belief that leather is a by-product of the beef industry and the skin would essentially be going to waste if it wasn't being used in clothing, as the cattle are being killed for their flesh anyway, meaning it doesn't have any significant ethical or sustainability impact. However, this is just a convenient way of attempting to rationalise something that is a core part of the overall problem. By this logic, the meat from dairy cattle would also be ethical and sustainable because the dairy cattle are primarily raised for their milk. Dairy farmers don't raise dairy cattle just for their meat, but that doesn't make eating dairy cows ethical or sustainable.

The key word is 'primarily'. After all, in the case of the meat for dairy farmers or the skin for cattle farmers, these additional products are still sources of income. In fact, while we might raise animals primarily for one product, we also use their bodies in a variety of ways to extract profit from them, from the gelatine we make from their bones to the fertiliser that we make from their blood, or indeed the clothes we make from their skin. While all of these extra uses are not the primary reasons the animals are raised and killed, or the primary revenue streams for those involved in the slaughtering, it all contributes to the continuation of these industries and the financial motivations of those involved. In the case of animal skins, leather can account for up to 26 per cent of the earnings of major slaughterhouses around the world.[3] So rather than viewing leather as simply a by-product, it should instead be viewed as a co-product and a significant part of the problem.

In fact, the price of cattle hides can decide whether or not a company is ultimately profitable. For example, a meat company in New South Wales made the news after it reported a loss of millions of dollars, with the biggest factor being that the price of cattle hides had dropped.[4]

To apply this argument to another situation, if a garment factory that exploited humans is always left with unused fabric after the garments have been made, would it be ethical to purchase it and provide them with extra profits just because this leftover fabric is not the primary reason the factory is in operation?

From a sustainability perspective, the issue with leather is not just the farming, but the post-slaughter processing too. Leather is chemically processed skin, because the hides of animals are not suitable for wearing unless they've been treated. According to the Leather Panel, which is part of the United Nations Industrial Development Organization, even if you only started counting after the slaughterhouse, the emissions associated with leather are higher than the total supply chain of producing artificial leather.[5]

Sometimes advocates of leather will claim that if we don't buy the leather, it will just go to waste, meaning that it is better to buy it than to not. However, again using data from the Leather Panel, as well as from other reports, it would be better from an emissions perspective to let the skin decompose in landfill than turn it into leather.[6][7] And this doesn't even take into account the water use, toxic eutrophication and more that comes with the processing of cow skin. Even if you factor in the production of synthetic leather on top of the emissions produced from sending the skin to landfill, it would still be preferable to producing leather. Plus, animal skins don't have to be discarded in landfills, as there are more environmentally friendly ways of disposing of them, such as composting them or turning them into biogas, which if used instead would make the alternatives even more of a sustainable choice. The animal farming sector chooses to discard the skins in landfills, which can negatively impact people's perception of synthetic leather by making it appear that the environmental impact of not using the animals' skins is higher than it needs to be.

All of this is also calculating the impact based on viewing leather as a by-product; however, as previously outlined, leather should be viewed as a co-product. This means that the impact of leather is even higher, as when the farming itself is also taken into account alongside the post-slaughter emissions, leather is responsible for nearly seven times the emissions of synthetic leather.[8]

Some advocates of leather point to vegetable tanning instead of using the chemical chromium as a more sustainable alternative. However, a study analysing leather-processing technologies found 'no significant differences' between the environmental footprint of vegetable and chromium leather-tanning processes.[9]

It's also important to note that synthetic polyurethane leather is not the only vegan alternative, or indeed the most sustainable. In fact, plant-based sources of leather are also where some of the most exciting forms of innovation are currently taking place within fashion and fabrics. For example, there are new leathers being made from cacti, mushrooms, kombucha, apple, pineapple and cork, to name but a few. There are also attempts underway to produce cell-cultured leather. While many of these products are not yet as widely available, the quality and commercial viability of new, innovative plant-based leathers are improving all the time.

Another interesting angle on leather is the difference in perception that exists around its origin and how it's produced compared to meat. One of the main arguments for eating meat comes from the idea of eating local or supporting British farmers, and while these ideas don't justify purchasing meat from UK farms, when it comes to leather, there is far less emphasis on even these ideas. In the case of leather, China is the biggest exporter, with Brazil coming second. However, China is Brazil's biggest importer of leather and so leather products made in China are also fuelling deforestation in Brazil. These products are exported all around the world and include footwear, bags, jackets, sofas, car seats and more. This applies beyond just products made in China though, as where a leather item is made is not necessarily the same as where the raw materials have come from.

One thing to look out for is when leather is used in smaller and less obvious ways. For example, jeans can sometimes have a leather patch, and leather can be used for specific elements of trainers, such as the tongues.

WOOL

Out of all the animal-derived clothing products, wool is often the one that causes the most confusion when it comes to why vegans don't buy products made from it. A huge part of this comes down to the perception we have of it and the marketing behind it. Wool is a product that has a long history in the UK, having formed a huge part of the economy in centuries gone by, and to this day it represents an industry that dominates our landscapes and reputation as a pastoral nation.

As a consequence, wool is viewed as a natural and ethical product that feeds into a wider narrative that we have in Britain about farming and land management. People often view wool as being a sustainable and ethical fabric, yet there's many reasons why this perception is worth scrutinising. To begin with, it is standard practice for sheep raised for wool to be slaughtered. The wool industry is a part of the sheep-flesh industry, meaning the same ethical problems associated with eating lambs apply to the wool industry too. The wool we wear comes from animals that are castrated, have their tails docked and have either already been or will at some point be slaughtered.

In the case of Australia, the world's largest wool exporter and the country where around 80 per cent of the world's merino wool is produced, lambs also go through a process called mulesing, which involves fully conscious lambs being restrained on their backs while flaps of skin are cut away from their tails and backsides. Mulesing is carried out to reduce the risk of flystrike, a condition where blowflies lay eggs in the folds of sheep skin and the subsequent maggots hatch and feed on the tissue of the animals.

The reason why mulesing occurs in Australia is down to a combination of factors. First, the merino breed that is favoured by Australian farmers has an especially large number of folds in their skin. On top of that, the climate in Australia is also ideal for blowflies, including the aptly named Australian sheep blowfly. Plus, mulesing is the most economical and hands-off solution for sheep farmers, providing a financial incentive. The fact that the merino breed continues to be used, despite the fact that it results in a process as brutal as mulesing, is down to the fact that merino wool can be sold for a higher price than other types of wool. There are also issues around the shearing of sheep, with exposés in countries such as the UK,[10] Australia[11] and New Zealand,[12] showing that abuse and cruelty can be found in the shearing sheds too.

Even the claim that wool is natural ought to be taken with a sizeable pinch of salt. While sheep do naturally produce wool, farmed sheep are selectively bred animals, and the wool goes through chemical processing, both of which do not occur in nature. In fact, the only reason that sheep produce excessive amounts of wool is because we have selectively bred them to do so. This is also why the claim that wool is ethical because sheep need to be sheared, which is one of the most commonly used arguments to justify producing wool, is not a strong one.

Sheep in the wild naturally shed their wool during the hotter months, which makes sense; after all, it's not as if for thousands of years humans have been wandering around with electric shearing clippers. It's also not the case that we acquire wool from animals in the wild who would die if we didn't shear them. We get wool by breeding animals into existence who have been selectively bred to produce huge quantities of wool. We then farm, mutilate, shear and slaughter them. This is not an industry that operates in the best interests of sheep, and it is certainly not an ethical one.

When we explore the realities that underpin these supposed ethical justifications, we can clearly see just how exploitative they are. We have selectively bred these animals in such a way as to maximise the profit we can extract from their bodies, even though the selective breeding comes at the detriment of their wellbeing. We then use the consequences of this selective breeding as a justification to continue exploiting and harming them.

The wool industry is therefore not a natural industry – instead, as is the case for animal farming in general, it is an example of humans hijacking natural processes and altering them using science and technology in order to make them better suit our desires and financial motivations. I would also argue that whether wool is natural or not is entirely irrelevant. The question is: is it ethical and sustainable? The answer is no on both counts.

So what about alternatives to wool?

One of the messaging points that the wool industry has used effectively is to draw a comparison between wool and polyester, making the claim that wool is a better product than a fabric derived from petroleum. However, this messaging is based on two false assumptions: one, that wool is more sustainable than synthetic fabrics; and two, that virgin petroleum-based fabrics are the only alternative.

In the case of synthetic fabrics, wool has been shown to produce more than three and a half times more emissions than nylon and nearly nine times more greenhouse gas emissions than polyester.[13] These figures are based on virgin fabrics; however, using recycled materials is also an option, meaning that wool alternatives can be produced from recycled polyester, which is commonly made from recycled plastic water bottles.

This false dichotomy of choosing synthetics over wool suggests that to avoid buying synthetic clothing you need to buy wool. However, this is clearly not the case. There are a variety of fibres that can be purchased instead, including hemp, cotton, lyocell (a fabric made from wood pulp) and bamboo. When analysing wool from Australia, the world's largest exporter, a wool knit jumper has been shown to emit 27 times more greenhouse gas emissions than a cotton one[14] and uses nearly 250 times more land.[15] When compared to lyocell, it is estimated that wool requires nearly 1,500 times as much land.[16] The issues related to synthetic fabrics do not then consequently justify the production of wool.

Importantly, in the case of leather and wool, these fabrics are produced from animals that are the least sustainable when it comes to the food that we get from farming them. We are routinely shown through the scientific literature that red meat is the most environmentally damaging food,[17] yet the systems of farming that produce these foods are the same systems of farming that produce the leather and wool products that we make from the same animals. Sadly, the wool industry is simply spinning a yarn when it comes to the claims that they make.

Outside of the more obvious woollen jumpers and knitted socks, wool is often used for suits and can be included in a garment as part of a mix of fabrics. So, even if a product is not obviously made from wool, it's always worth checking the label.

DOWN

Down refers to the feathers that are taken from ducks and geese. It is most commonly used as a lining in jackets and coats, as well as in pillows and bedding. All animals that are used for down are also slaughtered, and the production of down is inextricably linked to the intensive farming of these birds, with 80 per cent of down coming from China. It is also common for birds to be live-plucked, meaning the animals are pinned down and have their feathers roughly ripped off them.

Animal feathers can also come from animals who have been farmed for foie gras, an industry that is illegal in the UK. However, feathers from these industries can be imported into the UK, meaning that, similarly to fur, people are using a product that comes from a system that is not even legal in the country where they bought it.

Many companies will advertise that the down that they use is certified by the Responsible Down Standard (RDS). However, even though this is supposed to ensure that the birds were not live-plucked, Textile Exchange, who run the RDS, acknowledges that its standard 'might not guarantee 100% compliance all the time'.[18] Regardless, whether live-plucked or not, birds raised for down are raised and slaughtered in the same ways that birds raised for their flesh are. This also means that the sustainability issues surrounding intensive bird farming, such as feed use, waste and eutrophication, among others, are found within down production too, as are the use of antibiotics and the risk of viruses such as bird flu.

In the case of jackets and apparel, the most common alternatives to down are made by companies such as PrimaLoft, Thinsulate and Polartec. These companies make proprietary synthetic insulating materials, and they offer products made from recycled plastic and recycled fabrics. In the case of PrimaLoft, they also have a down alternative that biodegrades. Synthetic alternatives to down are also water-repellant, which down is not.

In the case of bedding, such as pillows and comforters, as well as synthetic materials, including the previously mentioned companies and their proprietary fabrics, there are also other products made from materials such as bamboo. Alternative fabrics to down are also used for anti-allergenic bedding, which can be especially helpful for people who suffer from ailments such as dust mite allergies.

SILK

Silk is the fibre that makes up the cocoons of silkworms. In nature, the silkworm goes through the same stages of metamorphosis – egg, larval, pupal and adult – that all moths do. However, the silk used in the fashion industry comes from domesticated silkworms that aren't allowed to go through all of their natural stages. Most of the insects raised by the industry are boiled, steamed or gassed alive inside their cocoons so we can use the fibre without damaging it.

Silkworms have also been selectively bred to have larger cocoon sizes and higher growth rates. Even though they have been bred this way, it is estimated that it still takes about 5,500 silkworms to produce 1 kilogram of silk. From a sustainability perspective, silk has been shown to have a significantly higher impact than other materials, including cotton and nylon.[19] Silk is also inefficient from a land use perspective due to the fact that silkworms only eat mulberry leaves. It takes at least 187 kilograms of mulberry leaves to produce 1 kilogram of silk, meaning that cotton production has a significantly lower water and land footprint compared to silk.[20]

As well as silk alternatives made from cotton and nylon, there is also lyocell and other fabrics. Plus, more innovative forms of non-animal silk production are also being developed. One example is Microsilk, which is a synthetic fabric produced by creating proteins that match those found in the silk of spiders.

THE FUTURE OF VEGAN FABRICS

Throughout this section on clothing, there has been a recurring theme. In much the same way that advocates for meat point to some of the aspects of plant farming that have environmental problems and use them to try and claim that animal products aren't as bad, advocates for animal-derived clothing do the same when it comes to certain materials that are suitable for vegans.

Synthetic fabrics such as virgin polyester are clearly not the best fabrics that we can or should be using, and they do of course have their own problems. However, the issues around these types of fabrics do not justify the use of animals for clothing, especially as the use of animals still brings with it a larger environmental and ethical footprint. Instead, the issues with certain synthetic fabrics should provide us with an incentive to opt for more sustainable fabrics and the motivation to revolutionise fashion in such a way as to create new, innovative and ultimately more preferable types of materials. Which is exactly what is happening.

The future of non-animal-derived clothing is extremely exciting, and there is a significant transition happening in the world of fashion. While cell-cultured meat is a more attention-grabbing technology, it is not the only development that is currently being worked on. From innovative plant-based leathers made from mushrooms, pineapples and apples to different types of wool and silk, the future of animal-free fashion is another example of the ingenuity and creativity of our species.

As well as transforming our food system, the way we produce clothing is also in desperate need of change. The fashion industry is far from perfect for a variety of reasons, including sustainability, human rights infractions and animal exploitation. Clearly there are still concerns around the production of fabrics that are suitable for vegans, including how our clothing is manufactured from a human exploitation perspective, as well as the general overproduction and overconsumption of clothes. The transition to a more ethical and sustainable model of fashion isn't, therefore, just about addressing animal exploitation. However, without removing the animal exploitation part, we will never be able to move to a fully ethical and sustainable system of production.

WHAT SHOULD I DO WITH CLOTHES I ALREADY OWN?
While veganism means no longer buying new clothes that are derived from animals, it is not so obvious what you should do with non-vegan clothing that you already own. Perhaps you have some leather shoes that you wear for work, or a winter coat that is lined with down, or a silk tie. The natural question then is: what should you do with these items?

This is another example of a grey area, as there is no hard-and-fast rule. It really depends on your situation and how you feel. For some people there are budgetary restraints that make buying a new wardrobe not possible, especially in the case of more expensive items such as winter coats. Certain items may have sentimental value, whether they've been passed down or are associated with a cherished memory. And if the items are still perfectly functional, some people choose to continue using them.

On the other hand, it is also very common for new vegans to look at their non-vegan clothes and feel uncomfortable with the idea of continuing to wear them. You might have a leather jacket and decide it just doesn't feel right to wear it any more, or a wool jumper that now reminds you of what happens to lambs and sheep. Some people are also of the opinion that continuing to wear your old non-vegan clothes contributes to the normalisation of wearing animal skins and wool.

While what you decide to do with the items of clothing you already own is a choice for you to make, one option I would recommend avoiding is just throwing the items away. If you decide that you no longer want to keep the animal-derived clothing you have, instead of simply putting them in the bin, consider donating them to a homeless shelter. This is especially important for items such as jumpers, coats and footwear.

Alternatively, some animal shelters will accept certain items of clothing, as they can be used for bedding. Or you could choose to sell them yourself and then donate the money to an animal sanctuary or an animal rights charity. That way you could stop someone from buying a new item and also raise some money to give back to benefit animals.

WHAT ABOUT SECOND-HAND CLOTHES?

The question of second-hand clothes is an interesting additional layer to the conversation around animal-derived clothing. After all, even if we recognise that buying animal-derived clothing is to be avoided, what about opting for second-hand animal-derived clothing over virgin fabrics suitable for vegans?

From a sustainability perspective, buying second-hand has obvious merits, even if that product would have had a large impact when it was first produced. And from an ethical perspective, the argument could be made that because the harm has already been done, buying a used item of clothing will be less harmful than buying something new, no matter what the material is. So what does this mean from a practical perspective?

First, the reason many vegans wouldn't want to buy these products is because they wouldn't want to wear them. Even if the justifications for doing so are not without their merits, the thought of wearing a second-hand leather coat, fur jacket or woollen jumper just wouldn't feel right, both literally and figuratively.

Second, the idea of buying pre-owned animal-derived clothing versus brand-new clothing presents a false dichotomy. Shopping second-hand is undeniably a great thing to do, but it's not just animal-derived clothing that is available. There are plenty of used clothes you can buy that are not made from animals, meaning that you don't have to choose between virgin non-animal fabrics and second-hand animal fabrics. However, that doesn't necessarily mean by default that buying pre-owned clothes made from animals is something to be avoided. So, beyond personal preference, are there any reasons why vegans shouldn't purchase second-hand animal-based clothes?

This is another example that could be considered to be a grey area. There are many vegans who are staunchly opposed to it and don't consider it vegan to wear these clothes, even if they are second-hand. They point to the fact that we wouldn't wear a jacket made from dog skin just because someone else had owned it before us, which means we are being inconsistent with our values if we then believe it is acceptable to wear second-hand cow skin.

Also, if you buy a pre-owned item of animal-derived clothing, it could be the case that you stop someone else from purchasing it who might then buy that item first-hand. In the case of a leather jacket, someone might have their heart set on one, find one in a thrift or charity shop and buy it. However, if you've already bought it, they might then decide to buy a brand-new one instead, thus contributing to all of the issues associated with the production of that item.

There's also the issue of whether wearing an animal-derived piece of clothing could make someone else see it and then want to purchase something similar, which would then have inadvertently contributed to more demand. And even if wearing something doesn't directly lead to someone else buying something similar, it does further contribute to it being normalised. In the case of something like leather, this might seem fairly arbitrary, considering leather is already extremely common. However, wearing a fur coat, which is far less common than leather and is not viewed as being socially acceptable in the same way, could normalise the idea of wearing fur.

In the interest of fairness, there is a crinkle in this argument: if products suitable for vegans are made to look like the product they are replicating, does wearing something that isn't obviously not an animal product also potentially normalise the wearing of the animal product it is replicating? For example, one time I was wearing a pair of vegan leather boots and in passing someone remarked to me that they liked them. My first reaction was to thank them for their kind words, but then I suddenly realised that I needed to tell them that they weren't real leather. So I quickly blurted out, 'They're vegan, actually.' In response, the person just nodded their head and said, 'OK.'

In that moment, I found myself stuck between a rock and a hard place – not say anything and run the risk of the person presuming they were real leather, or tell them and run the risk of the person thinking, *Why do vegans always have to tell people they're vegan?*

That being said, the use of non-animal alternative fabrics is extremely common now, particularly in the case of leather and knitted items, meaning that there might not always be an automatic assumption that an item is animal-derived. Plus, even if someone sees a pair of boots that they like and decide they want to get something in a similar style, many options available to consumers are not real leather, meaning that there's a good chance that the person might naturally opt for one of those anyway.

Another reason why vegans will often avoid wearing second-hand animal clothing is because it opens them up to being criticised and viewed as hypocrites, even if the item was pre-owned. One of my biggest frustrations when advocating for veganism is how quickly people try and find any sense of hypocrisy, and shoes have, in my experience, been one of the first places people look when it comes to searching for inconsistencies. For example, during an event I took part in outside of a rodeo in Texas, a cowboy, in response to me questioning him about the ethics of rodeo, looked at my feet and said, 'What about your shoes?' I then had to explain that my shoes were not leather. If they had been, even if they were second-hand, he would have felt vindicated.

His follow-up question was: 'What about your car? The seats are leather.' To which I had to explain that I didn't own a car. In the case of leather interiors for cars, the way of approaching it is more or less the same as it is for clothing.

Opting for non-leather interiors is the most ethical and sustainable choice – and in the case of second-hand, similar arguments around normalisation and influencing also apply. The opinion that it would be better to buy a used car with leather seats over a brand-new car with non-leather seats does have a lot of merit to it, especially when considering the wider impact of manufacturing a car beyond just the fabric used for the interior. However, if you are actively looking for a second-hand car, it's unlikely that the only options available will be ones with leather, meaning that it is probably not going to be the case that you will be choosing between a second-hand car with leather and a brand-new car without leather any way.

As you can probably surmise, the discussion around second-hand clothes is not quite as straightforward as the general conversation around animal-based clothing, hence why it is often viewed as a grey area. I personally do not buy used clothes that are made from animals for all of the reasons outlined. However, when it comes to going vegan, the most important thing is to avoid buying new clothes that are made from animals.

Entertainment

Animals used for entertainment has a particularly strong significance for me, as it was one of the big issues that led me on the road to veganism. Growing up, I was always fascinated by sharks and the oceans in general. A huge part of this fascination stemmed from my sense of fear around sharks and open water. As a consequence, I also found myself naturally drawn to movies about sharks, particularly the ones that depicted them as vicious and merciless killers. It must be said that the vast majority of these films range from truly awful to absolutely abominable. However, there is one very good one, which just so happens to be the one that started it all off: *Jaws*. I've always loved the film, although nowadays I do so with a significant pang of guilt due to the harm that both the book and the film caused to sharks, something that both the author of the book, Peter Benchley, and the director of the film, Steven Spielberg, later expressed regret about.

In the wake of the popularity of *Jaws*, another film came out that was ultimately less successful and is far less well known. Producer Dino De Laurentiis wanted to cash in on *Jaws*' success by commissioning a film with a similar premise but with some differences. One of those differences was that the film would be about another ocean predator, the orca.

Shortly after watching *Orca: The Killer Whale*, I saw a trailer for a new documentary that was coming out called *Blackfish*, which was about an orca that was being kept in an aquarium and had killed people. Considering my new interest in orcas as oceanic predators, this naturally piqued my interest, so I went to see the film.

It was genuinely horrifying, not because of the orca, but because of the humans. The film exposes the abject reality of aquariums and the immorality of confining animals that are then forced to perform tricks for our amusement. I saw the film and felt outraged by what was happening. As a consequence of seeing the documentary, I then joined a protest campaigning for the end of cetacean captivity.

Then, not long after seeing *Blackfish*, I went to Barcelona and visited the zoo there, where I watched a sea lion show. Upon seeing the trainers getting the animals to jump onto platforms and clap in order to be fed fish, I left the show as I realised that this was just another example of animals being exploited and demeaned for entertainment. These animals, who were already being held captive, were then being forced to engage in performances so that groups of humans could find some temporary amusement from their debasement.

After walking out of the show, I proceeded to wander around the zoo a little longer and came across a bear in an enclosure. The way the pen was laid out meant that I was looking down upon this bear, who was just sat on their backside by the wall. I suddenly felt so uncomfortable. Here was this animal trapped in this enclosure, with me literally looking down on them, and all for my entertainment. After watching this bear for some time and ruminating on how it was making me feel, I left the zoo.

While this didn't make me go vegan – I actually went and ate chicken for lunch after leaving the zoo – it was at this point in my life that I really started to think more about our relationship with animals and about the industries that I was supporting. All of a sudden, trips to aquariums and zoos, which had been among my favourite activities growing up, were off the table, as they caused me to feel extremely uncomfortable.

When it comes to entertainment, there are a number of different forms and types of events and venues to consider. The obvious ones include circuses, rodeos, bullfighting, dolphin swimming experiences and the aforementioned aquariums and zoos. While the use of animals for events such as bullfighting, rodeos and circuses is often viewed as immoral, many people who would never go to see a lion in a circus would go to see a lion in a zoo.

While it is unlikely that a book about how to go vegan will be read by people who don't see any issue with bullfighting and rodeos, the example of zoos is arguably more complex, especially if you are approaching a plant-based diet with the view of protecting the environment and think that a zoo's purpose is to carry out conservation work.

Undeniably, there are differences between lions in circuses and lions in zoos. In a circus, a captive lion is forced to perform and suffers repercussions if they do not, while a captive lion in a zoo is meant to be left more or less to their own devices. However, the reason people go to zoos is to see animals. Regardless of whether we perceive the performative aspects of zoos as being as overt as in other examples where animals are used for entertainment, people are still paying money to see a form of performance. This is why a common theme running through negative reviews of zoos is a sense of disappointment if the animals are not visible or are not engaged in interesting behaviour.

This sense of performance is also apparent when people try and get the attention of the animals or use flash photography. While this is often discouraged, and many people who go to zoos find it appalling when people do such things, this kind of behaviour is an extension of the mentality of entitlement and ownership that keeping animals in captivity for display purposes tacitly endorses.

For example, London Zoo hosts nighttime events with alcohol, food vendors and music. At these events, attendees often get drunk, which leads to people singing loudly, whooping and shouting, using flash photography, taunting animals and banging on glass. On one occasion, someone even cracked the glass of a reptile enclosure. There have also been reports of people trying to touch the animals and swim with the penguins, butterflies have been crushed, and during one evening someone poured beer on a tiger.[21] While London Zoo might not directly condone such things, it's naive at best not to think that after-hours parties with drinking and music would lead to drunken behaviour. London

Zoo stopped the events shortly after the 2014 report; however, they then restarted them later and claimed that the previous reports were 'heavily sensationalised'. At the time of writing, these events are still taking place despite the issues associated with them. London Zoo might argue that the funds raised from these events can be put towards their conservation work (more on that in just a moment), but even if this is the case, creating situations where the poor treatment of animals can ensue and even be made more likely is clearly not an acceptable way of raising money for other animals.

When it comes to circuses, we might think of animals being neglected or, worse, being physically and verbally abused and living under the spectre of fear-based control. With zoos, this is not the association we typically have, except for maybe so-called bad zoos. However, just because animals might not be treated as badly in one form of captivity compared to another does not then provide an ethical justification for the one that is not 'as bad'. And there are cases of comparable animal cruelty that have been documented taking place in some zoos. Moo Deng, a pygmy hippopotamus born in a zoo in Thailand, became an internet sensation after photos and videos of her were shared online. People flocked to see her by the thousands, doubling the number of daily visitors at the time. The zoo began selling merchandise and trademarked 'Moo Deng the hippo'. However, a handler at the zoo where Moo Deng was born had been filmed stabbing a baby elephant with a nail and using a bullhook handle. Elephants at the zoo are also chained and forced to do underwater performances where they swim, dance and do tricks. The zoo defended the performances by claiming that the shows should be 'considered exercise'.[22] Outside of the fact that Moo Deng is being exploited for the zoo's commercial interests, the zoo has used Moo Deng as a means to launder its image, even though its staff have been filmed doing things to animals that would be illegal in many countries and considered animal abuse. And it's not just in Thailand where animal cruelty has been documented. Animal abuse and neglect have been documented in other places, including Spain,[23] the UK[24] and Germany.[25]

Animals in zoos can sometimes develop zoochosis, which is a psychological condition in which animals kept in captivity display highly repetitive behaviours. This includes pacing, circling, neck twisting, head bobbing, weaving, swaying, rocking back and forth, self-mutilation and self-induced vomiting. The psychological impact of zoos is even acknowledged by the zoos themselves, as a survey of every zoo in the USA and Canada that housed gorillas found that half admitted to giving them pharmaceutical drugs such as Valium, Prozac and Xanax.[26] At a zoo in North America, a female gorilla was drugged with Prozac after she kept fighting off a male gorilla who was trying to mate with her. The drug was given until she stopped resisting him. These drugs, and others, have also been given to bears, chimpanzees, zebras, wildebeest and orangutans.[27] Animals in the UK have also been given antidepressants.[28] One researcher stated, 'At every zoo where I spoke to someone, a psychopharmaceutical had been tried.'[29]

Another study found that zoo elephants' lifespans were less than half of that of wild elephants in Africa and Asia,[30] and due to the ineffectiveness of captive breeding programmes, there have been more deaths than births within zoo elephant populations, meaning that European and North American zoo populations are not self-sustaining and are reliant on the capture of wild elephants. In fact, 75 per cent of female elephants over the age of 12 in European zoos and 80 per cent of female elephants over the age of 12 in US and Canadian zoos are believed to have been taken from the wild.[31] While there is a common belief that zoos no longer capture animals from the wild, this is not true and is still allowed, including, in certain circumstances, in the UK.[32]

In their defence, zoos position themselves as being essential for conservation. Some of the main ways that they claim to do so is through science, research and education outreach. However, before I discuss those, I want to focus on the most prominent aspect of zoo conservation, which is the breeding of endangered animals for re-homing in the wild. This is extremely misleading. There have been some cases of reintroduction of wild species using zoo animals, as was the case with the Arabian oryx and Przewalski's horse. However, these examples are few and far between and don't justify the confinement of every other animal species kept in zoos. After all, the captivity of elephants, lions, dolphins and bears had no bearing on the success of the Arabian oryx's reintroduction. This is because successful reintroductions require targeted breeding programmes. This is not something that we are reliant on zoos for, which is clearly demonstrated by the fact that the majority of successful reintroduction programmes have been carried out by government agencies and not zoos.[33] [34]

Releasing animals raised in captivity into the wild is also extremely difficult, especially in the case of large mammals. Fish, reptiles and amphibians can be reintroduced in a more straightforward manner, plus they can be far easier to breed. For example, frogs can be bred in huge numbers in a laboratory and released into the wild. However, these are not the animals most people come to zoos to see, nor are they the ones we think of when it comes to zoo conservation. Plus, zoos are not necessarily the place where these forms of breeding programmes are taking place, and it is also financially inefficient to run a whole zoo operation in order for a fraction of the revenue to go towards breeding a select few species of animals.

So if animals aren't being released into the wild, what happens to them? Back in 2014, the world looked on in horror as a perfectly healthy giraffe called Marius was killed at Copenhagen Zoo. However, he wasn't shot because he posed a threat to human life; he was shot because he was considered surplus to requirements. In other words, there were more giraffes than the zoo wanted. A few weeks later, the same zoo killed four lions, including two cubs, because they wanted to make space for a new male lion to use for breeding. This practice of killing healthy animals is not specific to just Copenhagen Zoo. It is conservatively estimated that every year up to 5,000 animals are killed by humans in European zoos alone. Why are these animals not being re-homed in the wild if this is supposed to be a core function of zoo conservation?

It is estimated that 70–75 per cent of the animal species in European zoos are not threatened in the wild, with only 5 per cent of mammal species and subspecies in European zoos being listed as critically endangered. Of all the species of animals held in European zoos, 95 per cent of them are not in captive breeding programmes, which means zoos are filled with animals that are simply being held captive – and even the species of animals that are in captive breeding programmes are not being bred with the intention of being released into the wild.[35] Instead, they are being held as an attraction to bring people to the zoo and as a reserve population for endangered species.

However, even if these zoos wanted to reintroduce animals into the wild, beyond the challenges of releasing animals who have spent their lives in captivity and who are not equipped to survive on their own, there's another problem. The viability of animals in captive breeding programmes is often jeopardised because of diseases, low levels of genetic diversity, hybridisation and inbreeding, meaning that mixing these animals with wild animals could weaken the genetics of the wild populations. In the case of London Zoo, a study showed that during the analysed period, two out of three lion cubs born there died because of the amount of inbreeding that had taken place. As one of the authors of the study put it, 'There are situations where they've bred the grandfathers with the granddaughters. This shows that the concept that zoos are conservation tools is completely false. This research blows that idea apart.'[36]

It is also contradictory that zoos talk about conservation and the current biodiversity crisis that exists while also serving animal products in their cafes and restaurants. This means that they are profiting from and continuing to perpetuate the industry that is the number one driver of biodiversity loss and species extinction both in the UK and indeed globally.

Although the breeding and reintroduction of animals is often viewed as the main way that zoos engage in conservation work, this isn't necessarily what the zoos themselves would claim. A report published by the Zoological Society of London, which runs London and Whipsnade zoos, states that 'most of the conservation activities carried out by EAZA [European Association of Zoos and Aquaria] member institutions do not relate to species reintroductions'.[37] Instead, zoos will often point out that they provide donations, grants and funding schemes to organisations engaging in conservation. However, in the UK, the British and Irish Association of Zoos and Aquariums states that 32 million people visit their members' zoos and aquariums every year.[38] They also state that their members contribute approximately £24 million per year to conservation projects.[39] This means that 75 pence per visitor is spent on conservation projects. Donating just £1 to these projects directly would therefore lead to more money being given to conservation.

Even when looking at the Consortium of Charitable Zoos, which is made up of nine members that run 13 zoos in the UK that are viewed as being among the best in the world, including London, Chester, Edinburgh and Whipsnade zoos, there are clear reasons for scrutiny. While these members promote that they provide conservation funding, it was revealed that at least 66 per cent of the total expenditure on conservation in natural surroundings came from grant income from external sources, with 80 per cent of one member's conservation expenditure coming from external grants.[40] This means that the majority of the money spent on in situ conservation is not even coming directly from the zoos themselves and has nothing to do with the captivity of animals. Some of these grants even came from government agencies, meaning taxpayers' money is being given to zoos, which are then passing the funds on to support conservation work and using this as positive PR for themselves.

When London Zoo spent £5.3 million on a new gorilla enclosure, the chief consultant to the United Nations Great Apes Survival Partnership said, 'Five million pounds for three gorillas when national parks are seeing that number killed every day for want of some Land Rovers and trained men and anti-poaching patrols. It must be very frustrating for the warden of a national park to see.'[41] One of Chester Zoo's most recent exhibits cost £40 million, which meant that it cost more than 26 years' worth of Chester Zoo's in situ conservation expenditure.[42]

Chester Zoo had an income of £57.4 million in 2023,[43] which is about the same amount as the annual expenditure of the Kenya Wildlife Service,[44] which manages 23 national parks, 28 national reserves and four national sanctuaries. They also manage four marine national parks and six marine national reserves. In other words, the income of just one of the more than 300 licensed zoos in the UK could fund the annual budget of the Kenya Wildlife Service.

The truth is that zoos use conservation as an attempt to make their captivity of animals seem more justifiable than it actually is. Zoos might have improved over time, but they exist now for the same reason they always have, which is to provide entertainment for people who are buying tickets to see animals in captivity. If a garment factory that exploited humans donated a tiny fraction of their revenue to human rights charities, would that make their exploitation of humans acceptable?

Zoos also claim that they serve as points of inspiration and get people interested in conservation. However, a review of a study that was initially carried out by the Association of Zoos and Aquariums stated that 'there remains no compelling evidence for the claim that zoos and aquariums promote attitude change, education, or interest in conservation in visitors'.[45] Plus, people have never seen animals like humpback whales or blue whales in captivity, and yet feel no less strongly about their protection than the animals they see in zoos.

It is true that many people who work in zoos care very much about the animals and are deeply worried about conservation generally. It is also true that zoos have been involved with and funded projects that have been beneficial for wild animals. However, the existence of zoos is not an essential part of conservation, funding or even breeding. In fact, zoos are inefficient in all these regards, and their existence causes unnecessary suffering and harm, and continues to normalise the idea that animals exist to gratify us.

While it might seem that there are no direct alternatives to zoos for vegans to engage in, that's not necessarily the case. Instead of viewing animals in captivity, we can instead go and see them in the wild. While African safaris and whale-watching experiences might not be possible for most people, observing animals can be as simple as going to a wildlife centre, such as an RSPB site or a national park. So if you are someone who is interested in animals and enjoys the idea of observing them, wildlife watching can be a really rewarding and enjoyable way of seeing animals, and on more mutually beneficial terms.

You can also visit wildlife sanctuaries created specifically to rescue animals, often from zoos, the irony being that these animals are moved to sanctuaries because they are unable to be re-homed in the wild. Many of these wildlife sanctuaries offer guided tours, although the main difference is that the sanctuaries exist to fulfil the best interests of the animals, meaning that the animals are given as much room as possible and privacy. You can also visit farmed animal sanctuaries, where you can spend time with cows, pigs, lambs, chickens and other domesticated animals.

There are also countless nature documentaries that allow us to watch and observe animals in far more interesting and informative ways than we can get in zoos and aquariums. While these animals might not be tangibly in front of us, the incredible craftsmanship that goes into making these programmes and the quality of the cameras used allows for a far more awe-inspiring interaction with these animals than watching them pace in circles or float in swimming pools.

Technology can also play a role in bringing us closer to animals. Virtual reality has the power to completely surpass any experience we could have with animals in captivity. Instead of seeing a lion in a cage, we could see a lion in their natural habitat and feel like we are there alongside them. Instead of watching an orca in a tank, we could be in the ocean with them. New technology has the potential to help us connect with animals in ways that most of us currently can't.

Toiletries, cosmetics and cleaning products

Animal testing for cosmetics and personal care items like shampoos and shower gels is one of the animal exploitation issues that people are most unified in their condemnation of. Even people who eat and wear animals still find themselves appalled at the idea that animals are used for testing. In fact, a survey carried out by YouGov found that nearly three-quarters of people in the UK oppose testing cosmetic products on animals, against just 9 per cent who support it.[46]

Fortunately, finding cosmetics and toiletries that haven't been tested on animals has become much easier over time. In fact, most brands that are cruelty-free will actively promote this on their packaging because it is a significant selling point. A really simple and easy way to find cruelty-free products is to look for the 'Leaping Bunny' logo, which is a certification given to brands that don't engage in animal testing.

In the UK, Superdrug has been approved by the Leaping Bunny programme, which means that all of its own-brand cosmetics and personal care range are certified cruelty-free. Plus, Boots, the other leading high-street cosmetics and personal care chain in the UK, has been certified as cruelty-free on more than 500 of its own-brand products. Not only is this great when it comes to the actual ethics of being cruelty-free, it also makes cruelty-free products affordable and very accessible as well.

One potentially confusing thing to be aware of, though, is the difference between cruelty-free and vegan. Cruelty-free refers specifically to whether or not the product has been tested on animals, but a cruelty-free product can still contain animal-derived ingredients, meaning that it's not vegan (or truly cruelty-free). One example of this would be a skin cream or moisturiser that came from a brand that doesn't test on animals but contains milk as an ingredient. This clearly wouldn't be suitable for vegans. As mentioned in the previous chapter, ingredients such as lanolin, shellac and carmine can also be used in cosmetics. So, as well as looking for a cruelty-free certification like the Leaping Bunny, it's important to check the ingredients list too.

If you use a particular brand, as well as checking on their packaging, you can also look online. If you're still unsure, or if they claim to be cruelty-free but don't have an official certification like the Leaping Bunny, you can always drop them an email and ask. The same is true for perfumes and aftershaves, which are other examples of common products that are not always suitable for vegans. While it is becoming increasingly common for fragrance companies to be cruelty-free, many still do not meet the criteria to be certified as such. Non-vegan ingredients can also be used by fragrance companies in their products, so it's a good idea to check to see if your favourite fragrances are vegan.

It's not just cosmetics and personal care products that can be tested on animals – cleaning and household products can be too. However, the same principle applies, as the Leaping Bunny programme also covers these products, and cruelty-free versions are easy to find in the UK. For example, leading retailers such as Sainsbury's, Marks & Spencer, Waitrose, the Co-op and Morrisons all have Leaping Bunny approval on their own-brand products.

Animal testing operates less on a supply-and-demand basis than other examples of animal exploitation. However, supporting cruelty-free brands will hopefully also incentivise companies that still test on animals to become cruelty-free as well.

Here is a list of common products that are sometimes tested on animals or contain animal products to keep an eye out for.

PERSONAL HYGIENE
- Toothpaste
- Soap and body wash
- Shampoo
- Conditioner
- Mouthwash
- Skincare products, such as moisturiser, sunscreen, eye cream, serums and acids
- Perfumes and aftershaves

HOUSEHOLD
- Limescale remover
- Bleach
- Surface cleaners
- Toilet cleaner
- Washing-up liquid
- Dishwasher tablets and rinse aid
- Laundry detergent and fabric softener

Medication

The other area in which animal testing takes place is medication and healthcare. While this subject is more ethically complex than the one around animal testing for toiletries, it is also far simpler in terms of what it means for vegans, because we don't have the choice between medicine that is and is not tested on animals. It is not a consumer-driven industry that operates on supply and demand, nor do we as consumers have a range of different products to choose from. This is not, therefore, an example of a grey area, as boycotting these medications is not a viable option.

I always feel really bad when vegans ask me if it's ethical for them to continue taking their medication, because nobody should feel guilty or question their morals for taking a medicine that they are reliant on. What happens during animal testing is the stuff of nightmares and horror films; however, even the strongest proponents of animal testing defend their position not because they necessarily believe it to be ideal, but because they believe it to be the best option available right now, although others would dispute this.

Thankfully, work is being done to shift away from animal testing, and there are non-animal technologies that are currently being used and that are in development. Plus, there is a general consensus that animal testing is ethically and scientifically far from perfect, meaning that even though we are still far away from eliminating animal testing completely, at least transitioning from animal testing is not as socially contentious or polarising as shifting away from animal farming.

Another aspect of medication that can prove to be ethically confusing is the use of animal-derived inactive ingredients that are used in the formulation of medicines. One of the most common is gelatine, which can be used in capsules and tablets. While opting for gelatine-free medication might not be possible for prescribed medicines, if you're purchasing over-the-counter tablets like paracetamol or cold and flu medicines, it is usually possible to find options that don't contain gelatine. For example, some medicines use pre-gelatinised starch instead of animal-derived gelatine, and you can sometimes find tablets that don't use gelatine or a gelatine alternative at all.

Another ingredient that can be found in medicines is lactose, which is derived from milk and can be used as a binder or as a filler for tablets and capsules. Similar to gelatine, it is normally possible to find over-the-counter medicines that don't contain lactose; however, the same is not necessarily true for prescribed medications. You can always ask your doctor or pharmacist if they have an option that is free from lactose or other animal-derived ingredients, but it is not guaranteed that it will be possible. The bottom line, though, is that you can only do your best.

That being said, shifting away from animal farming will naturally lead to changes in the use of animal-derived ingredients in other industries and sectors. If we are no longer exploiting and killing animals for food, then naturally we won't be using lactose and gelatine in medicines, as just from a purely practical and financial perspective, it wouldn't be possible.

As I mentioned right at the beginning of the book, veganism is not just a diet, and the practical aspects of being vegan go beyond just food. These other areas of veganism tend to be considered less, which is not necessarily surprising when you consider that food is a larger problem in terms of scale and is more challenging to address in terms of our own personal behaviours and choices. However, this does not reduce the importance of these other areas, or the problems associated with them. Whether it is clothing, toiletries, cosmetics or entertainment, hopefully you now know how to approach these changes too and what to keep an eye out for.

CHAPTER 5

NOW YOU'RE VEGAN, WHAT NEXT?

In previous chapters, I have covered behaviour change and how to succeed at going vegan, as well as all the different practical aspects of veganism and how to incorporate them into your life. However, once you've made the change, there are still several questions you might have or scenarios you might encounter. For example, you might be curious about the best way to navigate dating as a vegan, or what to do if you worry that you might have a nutritional deficiency. Some of the most common questions I get from other vegans are about children and pets, and whether they should be vegan too. In other words, there is much more to going vegan than what you consume and choose to purchase for yourself, and it is those aspects of going vegan that I address in this chapter. Many of these topics might come up for you immediately – if you are already in a relationship with someone, for example – whereas others might only become relevant for you a little further into your life as a vegan, in which case you can refer back to my advice in the years to come.

Let's start with the best way to approach a suspected nutritional deficiency.

What if I suspect I have a deficiency?

If we go through a period where we don't feel well, our automatic thought process can be to doubt the healthfulness of a plant-based diet. However, this thought process is not necessarily the same if we are just eating the standard diet that we have always eaten and that has less scrutiny around it.

This added attention doesn't have to be wholly negative, though, as it can provide us with a plan of action if we are feeling unwell. Many people who eat meat, dairy and eggs, and always have, might take longer to think about their diet as the cause. This could mean that a deficiency isn't picked up and that an underlying problem isn't addressed as quickly as it should be. On the other hand, the aforementioned scrutiny around plant-based diets could lead to us addressing any nutritional gaps more quickly and making changes to what we eat that safeguards us more in the future.

If you do notice that you are feeling worn out, less able to concentrate, or anything else that seems out of the ordinary, being mindful of the potential causes can be extremely helpful. There can be a multitude of reasons why we might experience periods when we feel under the weather. For example, are you feeling more stressed, or are you anxious or concerned about something? Do you enjoy your work, or do you feel overworked and burned out? How are you sleeping and are you getting enough rest? Are you exercising, drinking enough water, engaging in your hobbies? All of these, and more, can have a significant impact on our wellbeing.

This is why it's important to maintain a broad view of how we are living and taking care of ourselves. We could be eating healthily and nourishing our bodies, but if we are overworked or feeling stressed out, there's a good chance we are still going to feel depleted and worn down.

However, if you are feeling unwell and there isn't something else more obvious that is jumping out to you, then it could be worth tracking your food intake over a week and logging how much you're eating and the nutrients you are getting. That way you might be able to identify a pattern of something you are regularly missing out on. For example, if you can see that you are consistently not getting enough iron in your diet, making adjustments and incorporating more plant-based sources of iron could be something that might help (see the list of nutrients and key plant-based sources on pages 99–104). There are apps available that are specifically designed to help you analyse your nutritional intake, such as Cronometer – you just need to measure out the quantities of food that you are eating and add that information into the app.

Getting a blood test can also be extremely helpful if you are worried that you are feeling unwell, as the results will provide more clarity and understanding as to whether you are deficient in something. If you didn't have a blood test before you went vegan, you don't have a baseline to compare it to. In other words, you might have already been running low on a certain nutrient before you went vegan, and although your new diet hasn't made up for the deficiency, it is also not the cause of it. On the flip side, if you do have a pre-vegan baseline, you can easily identify if there is a nutritional gap in your new plant-based diet that can then be resolved.

In truth, having a baseline is really not necessary, though, as a nutrient deficiency needs to be resolved regardless. However, having a point of comparison can provide an extra element of context around the potential cause of any deficiency and how long it has potentially been around for.

If you've been living as a vegan and do find a nutritional deficiency, the question many people ask themselves is: should I go back to eating animal products?

If a meat eater is shown to have a vitamin B12 deficiency, for example, they will be told to take a B12 supplement. If a meat eater is found to have an iron deficiency and is anaemic, they will be recommended a form of iron supplement. While changes to diets are also recommended, those changes are tweaks rather than a complete overhaul. These changes also have to be made alongside wider health considerations. This is especially the case with regards to red meat, where general health guidelines are that we should be eating less, not more of it.

This way of dealing with deficiencies in meat eaters is the same approach we should have if we as vegans end up with any nutritional deficiencies. Rather than thinking that we need to go back to eating animal products, we should instead make sure that we are taking an adequate supplement and then make tweaks to our diet to ensure we don't have the same problem again in the future.

It's also important to note there are a number of reasons why nutritional deficiencies can occur outside of what we eat. You could be consuming a nutritionally well-rounded diet, but if you have an underlying issue such as absorption problems, a stomach ulcer or Crohn's or coeliac diseases you might see nutritional deficiencies anyway. So, if you are supplementing but the deficiency isn't getting any better, it might be that there is another underlying cause, in which case you should consult your medical practitioner.

Anyone, regardless of whether they eat animal products or not, can get nutritional deficiencies, but I hope that by reading this book you will be able to minimise the risk of developing any as a result of going vegan. However, if you do end up with a deficiency in an essential nutrient, the important thing to bear in mind is that this doesn't mean that a plant-based diet can't be healthy. Instead, it most likely means that you just need to incorporate a supplement to boost your levels,* make some adjustments and be mindful in the future that you are getting enough of the nutrient that you have become deficient in. That way you can continue to be vegan but also make sure that you are safeguarding your health.

Living with non-vegan friends

In Chapter 2, I discussed ways to communicate with your friends and family about your decision to go vegan. However, if you live in a flat or house share, there might be some other considerations to take on board.

Setting boundaries early on is really important, as that way you can avoid any potential sources of tension moving forward. For example, if the person you are living with asks you to buy something that's not vegan when you are going to the shop, this might not be something that you feel comfortable doing, especially if the expectation is that you're going to spend your own money. I believe buying animal products, even if they are for someone else, is something that should be avoided – after all, you've decided no longer to fund these industries.

The boundaries you set for yourself beyond this will be based on what resonates most with you and what your relationship with the people you live with is like. For instance, they might ask you to make something for them that contains an animal product, such as a cup of tea with cows' milk, and you might not feel comfortable doing so. Although you might be able to rationalise that you're not responsible for the harm that the purchase has caused, and the person you

---

* Many of the most common deficiencies that vegans are prone to are the ones that are covered by a vegan multivitamin.

live with is just going to make it for themselves anyway, it's still more than understandable if you don't want to be involved in that process. The problem is, even if you don't want to do it, you might feel a sense of pressure or expectation because you don't want to cause any problems and because you don't want to be seen as difficult.

Rather than doing something that makes you feel uncomfortable or running the risk of there being tension or an argument down the line, it is best to politely explain from the outset that while you're not stopping the people you live with from eating animal products, you personally don't want anything to do with them yourself, and this means not buying, cooking or using any animal products. If you can set that boundary early on, then moving forward you can remove the potential awkwardness or tension that can arise from being placed in a situation you don't want to be in.

Many vegans also don't like to cook using pots, pans and utensils that have been used to prepare animal products, so you might want to make sure that you have your own cooking equipment and that you explain to the people you live with that you would appreciate it if they would refrain from using it.

If you have shared ingredients and had a more communal approach to food in the past, it might also be helpful if you make sure that the people you live with don't use any food that you've bought specifically for yourself. That being said, if you have a good relationship with them, and they seem open-minded to making some changes, you could also suggest swapping certain household staples or foods that you communally share to ones that are plant-based. While encouraging someone to buy vegan over dairy cheese might not be possible, opting for plant-based spreads, stock, cereal, biscuits or breads, to name but a few, might be a suggestion that the people you live with are more receptive to.

When it comes to cleaning supplies and household products, suggesting some cruelty-free products – such as those that I mentioned in the previous chapter – is a simple way of making the products that are being commonly used more ethical, while also ensuring that everyone in the house can still use the same ones. Plus, because opting for cruelty-free household products is far less contentious than changing food, making these changes can be an easy and non-confrontational way of encouraging the people you live with to engage with the change that you have made and better understand it. These types of products could be a good starting point from which you can slowly encourage other changes within the household too.

You might also find that your boundaries change over time. At the beginning you might try and keep your veganism as close to yourself as possible so as not to ruffle any feathers or to create any extra barriers or struggles that could make the change more difficult for you. However, once you've become settled and confident in your veganism, you might then start to feel differently about how your interactions with others impact your principles and feelings. If you do find that your boundaries change over time, the important thing again is to communicate those changes.

One advantage of living with non-vegans is that it provides you with an opportunity to promote veganism by buying in plant-based products for people to try and by cooking plant-based meals for everyone you live with. Being vegan will naturally lead to conversations and discussions, so as well as there being difficulties associated with living vegan around non-vegans, it can also be a great way of bringing people together, and if the people you live with are positively influenced by you, it can even lead to stronger friendships and relationships as a consequence.

Dating as a vegan

If you are single, the question of dating as a vegan is clearly an important one – especially as dating can be a minefield even without veganism being added as an extra element.

As discussed throughout this book, veganism encapsulates a wide variety of different issues, and it is a reflection of our principles, values and beliefs. Sharing the same principles and values is one of the core ways of building a strong foundation in any relationship, especially a romantic one. This leads to many vegans feeling apprehensive about dating someone who isn't vegan, as they're worried that there will be a source of tension and disconnection that could jeopardise the long-term viability of the relationship. Also, many vegans don't want animal products in their house, so this can again be another source of disagreement and friction if you are already living with or move in with a non-vegan partner.

That being said, choosing only to date date vegans is not necessarily ideal. There are fewer vegans generally, and you might not live in an area where there are many vegans at all, let alone ones who are also looking for a partner to date. This can especially be the case if you are attracted to men, as statistically there are more vegan women than men.

The most important thing is to make sure that the person you are dating is not hostile, condescending or incredulous about you being vegan. This might seem like a fairly obvious thing to say; however, people do end up in relationships with people who are not supportive of their decisions or values. Not only is this a poor framework for a relationship, it can also lead to low self-esteem and people going back on their veganism so as to appease their partners. Many people who aren't vegan often perceive it as simply being a diet, and they might not, therefore, view it as something that is particularly important to you or that you are strongly committed to. Being upfront about your veganism from the outset means that the person you are dating understands its importance to you, and it also means that you can get a sense of the other person's opinions and views from the outset. It is understandable that you might feel apprehensive about how someone will react to you being vegan, and this might lead to you wanting to downplay it. However, doing so can lead to more problems in the future, and it might mean that you don't get a full understanding of the views that the person you are dating has.

Even if you find yourself a supportive and open-minded partner, there might still be some boundaries that you are not willing to cross and that they might not be aware of. One of the most obvious ones could be, as previously mentioned, paying for animal products for someone else. For example, you might start dating someone who isn't vegan and as a compromise go to a restaurant that has both vegan and non-vegan options. Perhaps on the first date the other person bought the meal, and now there is a pressure or sense of expectation that you are going to cover the cost of the meal for the second date.

This could clearly cause some problems, especially if your boundaries have not been communicated in advance. Not only can this have an impact on the date itself, it also means that you are making a situation more difficult for yourself – something that could have been avoided if your boundaries had been communicated earlier on and you had decided with your date that the easiest approach would be to split the bill. So if there are lines you would not want to cross – and not wanting to buy animal products is an extremely logical one considering you don't want to support the animal farming industries – then it's a good idea to make sure the person you are dating is aware of that before it could cause any issues. If you communicate your boundaries in advance, it also gives you the opportunity to work out any compromises. For example, if you want to treat your date, you could offer to take them to a vegan restaurant and pay for the whole meal. Alternatively, you could go out for drinks and buy some delicious vegan cocktails for them.

Dating can also be a great way of leading by example and positively influencing someone else to reconsider their choices and maybe even become vegan themselves. I know many vegans who started dating someone who wasn't vegan, and before long the person they were dating became vegan too. It should be said that dating someone specifically because it provides an opportunity to try and turn them vegan isn't an advisable or fair thing to do. However, if the person you are dating is accepting of your veganism and seems open-minded to it, that at least provides reassurance that you're not so dissimilar that a relationship isn't feasible, and it indicates that there is the potential that the person you are dating might one day go vegan too.

If you are looking specifically for another vegan to date, there are vegan dating apps available. Alternatively, going to vegan meet-ups, events and festivals can be a great way of meeting new people, making friends and potentially finding a vegan partner.

Living with a non-vegan partner

Deciding to go vegan can also have an impact on well-established relationships. If you are already in a relationship, it is equally important to be open and communicative. Your partner is probably unsure of how you going vegan will impact their life, so being able to explain what it will practically mean for them is vital. This will be especially the case if you live together, as food shopping and cooking will be affected.

Hopefully, your partner will be on board and supportive, and even if they don't want to go vegan themselves, they'll be accommodating and eat plant-based meals with you. However, if at first your partner seems disgruntled and unhappy about you becoming vegan, then it's important to be patient and understanding. This is a change that affects them too, and they may feel unsure or worried as to what it will mean for them and for your relationship. You should listen to your partner's concerns and see if you can work together to address them, while ensuring that you are not compromising on your choice to become vegan.

Setting and communicating boundaries is again really important. Your partner might also want to set boundaries with you regarding what they are willing to do, so finding workarounds and compromises is key. I know vegans who are dating someone who isn't vegan and their non-vegan partner eats vegan at home but will eat animal products if they are at work or socialising with friends. Alternatively, if that's not a workable compromise and they want animal products in the house, can they accept that you won't want to buy or cook any of them?

Outside of food, setting boundaries around other aspects of veganism is important too. For example, if you used to go to zoos or aquariums when you visited different cities on holiday, making sure your partner knows in advance that this is something you no longer want to do is important. Likewise, if your partner has a track record of buying you clothes as presents, then making sure they are aware that veganism also means abstaining from purchasing animal-derived clothing means you don't have to worry about being given a present that is made from animals.

If your partner is initially resistant to you going vegan, they will hopefully become more accepting and supportive over time as they get used to what it means and adapt to the changes that have taken place.

One big consideration around having a non-vegan partner is children. If you already have a long-term partner or you start dating someone and the conversation of children comes up, it is again incredibly important to discuss it in advance so that you are both on the same page about how your children will be raised.

Raising vegan children

Vegan children can be a very emotive subject, and people don't always approach it with the level of rationality or understanding that they should. But even though the topic of vegan children still remains fairly controversial, from a nutrition and health perspective it is entirely possible. For example, the British Dietetic Association states that 'carefully planned plant-based diets can support healthy living at every age and life stage'.[1] The NHS also supports the claim that a plant-based diet can provide all the nutrients a child needs, as long as parents ensure that they provide enough energy and vitamins for any babies or children they are raising vegan.[2]

Of course, this is true of all parents, regardless of the type of diet. No diet automatically guarantees that a child won't become unhealthy and suffer from malnutrition. A child raised on an omnivorous, pescatarian, vegetarian or plant-based diet can end up lacking essential nutrients if their parent or caregiver isn't giving them everything that they need. Any diet requires knowledge, preparation and care – and it is the responsibility and moral duty of a parent to ensure that they are taking proper care of a child whether they're vegan or not.

Cases where children raised on diets free from animal products suffer from malnutrition or die never fail to make the news. However, when they do, the issue tends to be framed around the fact that the parents didn't feed the child any animal products. What consequently happens is that a plant-based diet is blamed alongside the parents for being responsible for the child's death. However, when an omnivorous child suffers from malnutrition or dies, the messaging is never that there is something fundamentally wrong with eating animal products. The responsibility for the child's death is placed solely on the parents or caregivers.

Sadly, this discrepancy in reporting perpetuates the narrative that plant-based diets are inherently dangerous for children, when this is not true. Instead, these cases tend to involve parents who were feeding their child clearly unhealthy diets; for example, in 2019, an 18-month-old child died after being fed only raw fruits and vegetables. This case was covered internationally, with the phrases 'vegan mom' or 'vegan couple' used throughout the reporting.[3] But whether or not the parents were vegan isn't the important aspect of this case or others like it. What is relevant is that they only fed their child raw fruits and vegetables.

It's important to clarify this, because much of the conversation around plant-based diets for children centres around the question of whether or not it is a viable option, even though the experts have said that it is. Sadly, headlines, stories and negative conversation about raising children vegan can lead to vegan parents second-guessing themselves.

As soon as we acknowledge that it is possible to bring up a child on a vegan diet, we can address the more important question of how to do it. This reframing can also be incredibly valuable, as it can alleviate any doubts about the overall viability of a plant-based diet for children – as can recognising and reminding ourselves that our leading health authorities also support that a plant-based diet can be healthy. The onus is then on parents to ensure that they are giving their children all the nutrients they need. Thankfully, there are lots of great resources online that you can consult, a selection of which you can find in the Resources section of this book. Similarly to adults, the key nutrients to look out for include vitamin B12, calcium, iron, vitamin D and iodine. If your budget allows, you could also consider working with a registered dietitian.

One really important aspect of the conversation is baby formula. If breastfeeding is not an option, using formula milks is the only alternative that will ensure that a baby is getting all of their nutritional requirements. There are some accredited vegan formulas on the market, but these are not always widely available, although they can often be ordered online. It's incredibly important that a proper formula is used, so don't opt for regular plant milks from supermarkets or a homemade formula. If it's not possible to get a completely vegan formula, then just opt for whatever the best accredited formula option available to you is.

One of the biggest criticisms of raising children vegan is that parents are forcing their child to be vegan or pushing their values onto them. However, a child is unable to make these decisions for themselves, so any diet is decided for the child by the parent. If a parent's values mean that they perceive eating animals to be moral, then by feeding their child animals, they are also pushing their values onto their child.

Plus, the animal products parents feed to their children are based on what is culturally normal. This means that by feeding our children some animals and not others, we are simply forcing what is culturally normal onto our children. So, if you are accused of forcing your views onto your child, or if someone claims it is unethical to raise a child vegan, try not to take it to heart, although I appreciate that this can be easier said than done, especially if it is coming from within our families, such as from our parents, in-laws or siblings.

If you do find that your family have any concerns or worries, it's important to understand that these are more than likely coming from a caring place. Having a response to any questions they have is not only a good way of trying to alleviate their worries, it also means that you are more informed and knowledgeable too. If you can explain to them why you have made the decision, how our leading health authorities support the fact that children can be healthy vegans, and why any criticisms related to forcing your views on them are invalid, that could help allay their concerns and mean that you start receiving fewer comments or criticisms. However, this might not always be possible, in which case it's important to remember that the views and opinions of others are not your responsibility. As long as you are raising your child healthily and responsibly, then that's what matters the most.

And if you do find yourself on the receiving end of any criticism, then hopefully the longer your child is vegan and healthy, the less criticism you will receive. Plus, the more normal raising vegan children becomes, the easier it will become. I know many vegan parents who have raised their children vegan and have found it far simpler and more widely accepted than they were anticipating.

But what if you already have children and want to transition them to a vegan diet? If you're going vegan on your own, and your partner isn't going vegan with you, there might not be any significant change for your child when it comes to you going vegan. However, if you're a single parent, or if your partner is going vegan with you or is happy to only have plant-based food in the house, then that will have more of an impact on your child. How much of an impact will completely depend on the age of the child or children you already have. If your child is young enough that you still make all the decisions for them in terms of what they eat, then it makes sense to transition them to plant-based food too. Even if they are young, explaining to them the reasons that you've gone vegan and communicating what this will mean in terms of the food they are eating could be really helpful for them, as it will allow them to have a better understanding of what changes are happening and why. Children often have greater clarity when it comes to animals, and while it wouldn't be appropriate to show them upsetting footage or to discuss with them the more violent aspects of animal exploitation, framing your decision more broadly as being about compassion, kindness and empathy for animals can be a really effective way of broaching the conversation with them.

With young children, they might go to birthday parties for other children, or they might be in environments where foods containing animal products are offered to them. How you choose to handle these situations is entirely up to you. I know vegan parents who will buy a vegan cake that their child can take to a birthday party so that they have something to eat when all the other children are eating the non-vegan birthday cake. I also know vegan parents who take a more relaxed approach and allow their children to eat the non-vegan birthday cake because they don't want their child to feel like they are different, especially if the child might not be old enough to fully understand the situation and why they are eating something different to everyone else.

If your child is older and goes out with their friends and is in situations where they make choices and decisions for themselves, then how you approach veganism with them will vary depending on how receptive or open to it they seem. I've met vegan parents whose children also went vegan of their own accord. I've also met vegan parents whose children still eat animal products because they didn't want to change when their parents did. There are a number of reasons why a teenager might not want to follow what their parents are doing, and it's important to be understanding and empathetic towards them. For example, they might be worried that they will get teased or bullied at school or by their friends.

As they're older, you could have a more in-depth discussion with them about the ethics of what we do to animals. If your initial inspiration to go vegan came from a video or documentary that you watched, depending on the contents, you could encourage them to watch it too so that they gain more insight into your rationale.

Even if your child is accepting and supportive of you going vegan, they might still not want to do so themselves. This means that when they are in situations where they are choosing their own food options – such as when they're out socialising – they might still decide to consume animal products. While discussing these choices with your child is a good idea, arguing with them or demanding that they comply with your wishes could lead to a disconnection and to your child simply not being honest with you or talking to you about what they're doing.

This is clearly not ideal for a number of reasons, and arguing over their choices is probably just going to push them further away anyway. This is especially true if they're at an age where they might be more inclined to be rebellious and are trying to find out more about themselves and their own identities. Instead, validating any concerns they have and offering them the space and autonomy to make their own choices is a good way of allowing them to get to grips with veganism in a more appealing manner. You can also use the fact that you are vegan to positively influence them by cooking them delicious plant-based food, getting them vegan versions of their favourite foods so that they can try them themselves, and living by example. Even if your child doesn't want to go vegan with you at the beginning, approaching the change with them in this way will hopefully mean that they view veganism more favourably, and that they come around to the idea in time once they've had an opportunity to understand what it actually involves and have got used to you being vegan.

Ultimately, when it comes to family and children, it's impossible to have a one-size-fits-all solution. The bottom line is again to do what you can. Living vegan yourself is the most important aspect of all of this. If you can encourage others to do the same, or to eat more plant-based meals, then that is wonderful. But if that's not possible, just do your best. As long as you don't allow the choices of others to make you feel negatively about yourself, or to impact your conviction, then that is the main thing.

What about pets?

As well as partners and children, there's also the question of pets – or, as I like to call them, companion animals. Maybe you already have a pet, or maybe you've gone vegan and are wanting to get a companion animal but are not sure how to go about it or what you should feed them.

Let's start with the scenario that you've gone vegan and now want a furry companion to hang out with. When it comes to pets, the golden rule of doing so ethically is to adopt not shop. In the UK, and around the Western world generally, we condemn the abuse of dogs and cats, and sign petitions calling for the end of people eating these animals. However, even where we live, dogs and cats don't escape from our exploitative and harmful behaviours.

It is estimated that more than 100,000 dogs and more than 1 million cats are either in shelters or are strays in the UK.[4] It is also estimated that around 20,000 dogs are put down every single year, with Battersea Dogs and Cats Home reportedly euthanising 27 per cent of the dogs they take in.[5]

Upon hearing this, many people's first reaction is to condemn the shelters and rehoming organisations. However, while euthanising healthy animals is far from ideal, if these animals have behavioural issues because they've not been raised or looked after properly, or nobody is rehoming them and they are just being left in a kennel, meaning other animals are unable to be rescued, what is the alternative?

No-kill shelters sound better, but looking after these animals costs money, and they are often kept in small enclosures, which can lead to a poor quality of life. Plus, once a no-kill shelter is filled with animals that can't be re-homed, what happens to all the other stray, abandoned and relinquished animals?

Shelters are a symptom of a wider problem, and pointing the finger at shelters just distracts from the real culprits – mainly, breeders. Opting for animals from breeders perpetuates the problem of homeless animals. And because commercial breeders do what they do for money, by purchasing a puppy or kitten from them you are incentivising them to breed more puppies and kittens.

Animals from breeders can also be prone to health problems, birth defects and incorrect medical care. Many breeders also opt for popular breeds who have been selectively bred in such a way that causes them suffering and hardship. These ailments include dislocated kneecaps, heart problems, skin and eye infections, heart attacks, hip dysplasia and the list goes on.

The most obvious of these problems can be found in dogs that have been bred to have flat faces and shortened skulls, such as pugs, French bulldogs and boxers. Breathing for these animals has been described as being like inhaling through a straw, leading to them panting and gasping to get enough air. This also impacts their ability to regulate body temperature, leading to heatstroke. Pugs can also suffer from pug dog encephalitis, which is a fatal brain disease.

Societally speaking, we call ourselves dog lovers while breeding some breeds of dogs in such a way that makes their lives worse, and we do it because we think it makes them look cuter. We are reducing their quality of life so that we can derive a slightly higher level of pleasure from their appearance. Even if buying from a commercial breeder was ethically justified, buying these types of breeds would still be wrong. In fact, countries including the Netherlands, Austria, Germany and Norway have banned or restricted the breeding of breathing-impaired breeds. In the UK, the British Veterinary Association has also called for people to choose different breeds.[6]

If you already have a dog who suffers from any of these problems or is one of these breeds, then this is clearly going to be deeply upsetting. However, outside of potentially being more mindful on particularly hot days, this shouldn't mean that anything changes when it comes to you caring for them. Becoming vegan can mean discovering or thinking about things in ways that we might have not done previously. While this isn't always pleasant, it is not a negative reflection on us if we become aware of new information that might lead us to make different choices in the future. This is in essence the crux of becoming vegan, as it's not about chastising ourselves for our past choices, but instead about learning, developing and making different choices moving forward.

Another important consideration when looking to get a companion animal is understanding how to properly train and look after them. People often underestimate the time and commitment required, or don't realise just how big of a responsibility having a pet is. This can lead to people deciding to get rid of the pet, which can include sending them to a shelter or, in more extreme examples, abandoning them.

There is no better example of this than during the Covid-19 pandemic. Due to lockdown and working from home, millions of households in the UK acquired a pet. However, by the end of 2022, with the pandemic easing, people returning to work and a cost-of-living crisis severely impacting society, the number of animals being abandoned started to increase. In 2024, both Cats Protection and the RSPCA called the levels of pet abandonment and animals in shelters a 'crisis'.[7] Many of the puppies bought at the beginning of the pandemic were also not properly socialised with other humans or dogs, leading to behavioural problems.

Another important consideration is sterilisation. Even though the UK has higher rates of sterilisation compared to other countries, pets can breed at a rapid rate, which can lead to more unwanted animals. This is especially important with cats, who are generally more independent and also make up the majority of stray animals.

Adopting an animal rather than buying one might mean that it's not always possible or easy to get the exact breed that you'd ideally like, or to have a newborn puppy or kitten. However, it's important to evaluate what the intention behind having a companion animal is. If you want a pet because you want to give an animal the best life possible, and you want to have a non-human friend who you can hang out with and develop a bond with, then adopting is an amazing way of giving an animal a life that they wouldn't be able to have otherwise.

The same applies to pets who are not dogs and cats. Rodents and other animals are commonly bred for the pet industry in breeding centres, also known as rodent mills. These operate on the same principle as puppy mills (or animal farms more generally, for that matter). These animals are bred for profit, and investigations have revealed that these facilities are essentially factory farms for pets.[8] There are a number of organisations and shelters that also rescue smaller animals, meaning that you can also adopt rabbits and rodents (see the Resources section).

PLANT-BASED DIETS FOR PETS

If you already have companion animals in your life, depending on the species, you might find yourself querying whether they should be eating a plant-based diet too. In the case of rabbits and rodents, the answer to this is fairly straightforward. However, what about cats and dogs?

The first thing to recognise is that our furry friends also have a climate pawprint that needs to be addressed. In the USA for example, it is estimated that pets consume a third of the meat that humans consume,[9] and it is estimated that as much as 20 per cent of meat and fish is consumed by pets globally.[10] This is especially problematic if people are feeding their pets meat that is intended for human consumption, which has the equivalent ethical and environmental impact that humans eating meat does. In fact, if the production of dry cat and dog food in the USA used meat that was originally intended for humans and is not considered to be by-products, this would mean between 25 per cent and 30 per cent of the emissions associated with animal products in the USA would be attributed to pets.[11]

However, pet food is usually made from by-products. These have a lower economic value, which means that their environmental impact is not as high relative to the economic value of the products. Even when taking this into account, the global production of dry pet food still has a land footprint of more than twice the area of the UK, and the greenhouse gas emissions produced would rank dry pet food as having a greater impact than more than two-thirds of countries globally.[12]

More importantly, the revenue generated by the sale of by-products further continues the animal farming industries as a whole. According to a published article on pet food by the National Renderer's Association, 'The sustainability of animal agriculture depends on a reasonable and practical use of the by-products generated.'[13]

All of this leads to the ultimate question: what should we feed our dogs and cats? The British Veterinary Association has stated that it is possible to feed dogs on a plant-based diet,[14] and there is some early evidence that indicates that dogs could even be healthier when put on plant-based diets.[15] Add to this that a systemic review of the scientific literature so far on plant-based diets for dogs and cats found that 'there is little evidence of adverse effects arising in dogs and cats on vegan diets', although they also stated that 'a cautious approach is recommended'.[16]

Even though raw-meat diets for dogs are often viewed as being culturally more acceptable, they pose a greater health risk when it comes to the spread of pathogenic and zoonotic bacteria. Research papers have even warned that feeding dogs raw meat may be fuelling the spread of antibiotic-resistant bacteria. In one example, an outbreak of E. coli in England in 2017 led to four people becoming infected, three of whom were children, with one person dying. At least three of the cases came from exposure to dogs who were fed on a raw-meat diet.[17]

A study by the University of Bristol found that 87 per cent of raw-chicken dog food was contaminated with E. coli that was resistant to certain antibiotics, and nearly half of the chicken was contaminated with E. coli resistant to fluoroquinolones, which are a type of antibiotic that the World Health Organization has classified as being 'critically important' to human healthcare. A similar amount of resistance was also found in raw chicken meant for human consumption.[18] However, while still posing a risk, humans cook raw chicken and tend to have higher hygiene standards when preparing their own food. Not only can raw meat contaminate anything that it comes into contact with – including anything the dog then licks after eating the meat – but the bacteria can also be excreted by the dog later. This means there are multiple risk factors involved and more potential routes through which the bacteria can spread.

While dogs can eat home-cooked food, ensuring that nutritional requirements are met is not necessarily easy, especially as the ratios of different nutrients differs for dogs compared to humans. This is why buying a plant-based dog food is a safer and simpler option. If you already have a dog and are interested in transitioning them to a plant-based diet, there are a growing number of dog-food options. Make sure the one you get is listed as being nutritionally complete. It could also be advisable to incorporate the plant-based food over time, rather than completely switch overnight.

You could also take your dog in for a health check before you start the transition and then again after a period of time to see how their health compares. Not only will this give you peace of mind, it also means you can make any adjustments. As discussed previously in the chapter, getting a baseline can be helpful. If your dog has a deficiency or something wrong with them, a plant-based diet could be falsely blamed if whatever's wrong is only detected after they've made the transition. Alternatively, if there is nothing wrong with your dog beforehand, that means if anything is picked up at later check-ups, you can more easily identify if it does have anything to do with their plant-based diet.

The conversation around cats is more controversial, and understandably so. Even in vegan forums this can be a hotly debated subject. Cats in the wild are obligate carnivores, meaning they need to eat meat to survive – or, more specifically, they need certain nutrients, such as taurine and vitamin D, that, in the wild, can only be obtained from meat. This distinction is important, as it signifies that it's not the meat that is necessary, but what is in the meat. In theory, this means that if the food had these nutrients in it and to the right levels, a cat could be healthy on a plant-based diet. Commercial cat food is commonly fortified with these nutrients. So, if feeding a cat meat that is fortified with essential nutrients is viewed as being a healthy option, it then follows that feeding a cat something that is not meat but that is fortified with the nutrients the cat needs can be healthy for them too.

One of the arguments people like to use in favour of meat-based diets for cats is that it's not natural for them to be eating plant-based diets. However, it's not natural for them to be eating beef or tuna either. After all, the likelihood that a domestic cat is going to bring down a cow or swim into the Atlantic Ocean and catch a tuna is much lower than them eating something from a plant. That being said, domesticated cats do catch and kill birds and small mammals, but these are not the animals that we feed to them, and nor should we start doing so, as this would mean increasing animal suffering and the number of animals being killed.

This touches on an important ethical consideration: how do we value the life that is taken to sustain the life that we are caring for? If there is no moral difference between the life of a pig, cow or lamb compared to a cat, then to contribute to the deaths of these animals to feed a cat over their lifetime poses a significant ethical dilemma.

Some vegans I know opt to feed their cats fish, believing this to be a more ethical compromise. However, this is based on an assumption that fish suffer less, which we don't know to be true. Plus, feeding cats fish actually leads to more animal deaths, and because of what happens to both farmed and wild-caught fish, it could increase the overall amount of suffering involved too. There's also the significant environmental harm from fishing and fish farming to take into consideration.

So, using pet food that utilises the less desirable parts of rendered animals would appear to be more ethical, with beef options arguably being the best from a suffering and death perspective. However, cattle farming is the most environmentally harmful, so there's a dilemma there too. And, as previously mentioned, the pet food industry is a valuable revenue stream for the animal farming sector, meaning that even these types of pet foods are still contributing to an industry that we recognise as being immoral and harmful.

With all this in mind, if we can make sure cats are healthy and well cared for, while at the same time not contributing to the exploitation and harm of animals in farms, then that would be ethically and environmentally preferable. In other words, if a plant-based diet is possible for cats, then the merits for it are clear.

Some might claim that feeding raw meat to cats is a natural option, but not only is this not a strong argument, it also comes with considerable risks. For example, an outbreak of bovine tuberculosis in cats in the UK in 2019 that was traced back to a commercial raw-venison cat-food product had a mortality rate of 83 per cent in the cats who were initially reported as becoming sick,[19] and there were some reports that it may even have infected four owners and one veterinary surgeon with latent tuberculosis.[20]

In reality, there is nothing natural about having domesticated and selectively bred animals living in our homes and eating other domesticated and selectively bred animals, or fish caught out at sea or farmed in pens. The animals we have in our homes are not natural animals, and their diets and lifestyles are not natural either, regardless of whether they eat meat or not.

Unfortunately, just because something is possible in theory does not mean that it is possible in practice. Plant-based cat food is not as widely available, and cats are fussy eaters – if you have a cat that is used to a specific type of food, they might not want to eat a new one. It is also the case that cats can have varying needs, with vet-prescribed or specialised diets sometimes being required.

It is also important to state that, at the time of writing, the British Veterinary Association has not yet taken the position that plant-based diets are suitable for cats. This might change in the future, like it has with dogs. However, the trade organisation UK Pet Food, which creates guidelines for pet food, believes that plant-based diets for cats can be suitable.[21] They highlight that there are products available on the market that you can buy, but you need to make sure that you choose one that is nutritionally complete. Just as with dogs, it is not advisable to feed cats home-made diets, whether plant-based or not. When it comes to cats, home-made plant-based diets will almost certainly lead to nutritional deficiencies.

It's also worth noting that getting nutritionally complete cat and dog food is not necessarily a certainty when it comes to meat-based food either. A study in the UK found that only 30 out of the 80 dry foods that were tested were fully compliant with EU guidelines, and only 6 out of 97 of the wet foods were compliant. Many of the products tested were shown to have excessive or insufficient levels of nutrients. These foods, if used over a prolonged period, could contribute to a whole host of health problems, including dermatological, skeletal and neurological diseases. The study also showed that foods with high fish content, particularly for domestic cats, had high levels of undesirable metal elements such as arsenic.[22]

There are meat-based pet foods that are not nutritionally complete, and there are plant-based pet foods that are nutritionally complete and compliant with guidelines. So, even though the perception is that plant-based diets for cats are lacking nutrients, a vegan feeding their cat nutritionally complete and compliant plant-based food is arguably going to be ensuring better nutrient intake for their pet than people who are feeding incomplete and non-compliant meat-based food. The bottom line is, regardless of which diet you feed your cat, make sure the food you choose is nutritionally suitable, as it's not necessarily a given.

If you are thinking of incorporating plant-based food into your cat's diet, regular health check-ups are necessary. And, as mentioned before, getting a baseline health check can be really valuable. It also doesn't have to be an all-or-nothing type of approach – you could mix some plant-based cat food into your cat's regular diet and see if they enjoy it.

The good news is that cell-cultured meat is perfect for the pet-food industry. It removes the potential controversy of plant-based diets for cats and also dramatically reduces the ethical and sustainability problems with pet food and meat. On top of that, cell-cultured pet food went on sale for the first time in the UK in early 2025, meaning that it should hopefully not be too long before cell-cultured pet food becomes widely available.

Alternatively, if you're looking to rescue an animal and you don't have access to a nutritionally complete plant-based cat-food option, there are always rabbits that need rescuing.

CHAPTER 6

HOW TO BE VEGAN IN A NON-VEGAN WORLD

Before I was vegan, I saw the world very differently to how I see it now. There was a time when I would walk through a supermarket and not think twice about the rows of body parts that lined the shelves. When the red glow from a butcher's shop window and the pungent smell that drifted out didn't cause me to stop and think of the animals whose flesh was there on display. When a cow was just a cow and not a mother. When chicken came fried in a bucket, not from an animal who had lived a wretched life and suffered a terrifying death. And there was a time when a zoo was a fun day out, horse racing was entertainment and leather was just a fabric used to make clothing. Going vegan has changed all of that.

Now, when I travel through the countryside, I notice buildings that have always been there but that I never saw before. Buildings that bear no markings yet sit nestled among the landscape. Salient yet unnoticed. Conspicuous yet ignored. These buildings are everywhere, and millions of animals are locked inside these prisons. Yet their persecution doesn't exist because of any wrongdoing on their part, but simply because they were unfortunate enough to be born into the body they were born into. They are simply the unlucky ones.

However, this isn't a system that runs on luck. This is a system that deliberately breeds animals into these environments. It is an inherently cruel and exploitative system that by its very nature should expose itself as being profoundly wrong. A rigged system interested only in maintaining the privileges and power of those it benefits, with no regard given to those who are harmed as a consequence.

Perhaps most jarring of all, I now notice the trucks driving on motorways. Huge vehicles filled with animals who are being taken to slaughterhouses where their lives are going to be extinguished. The enjoyment of a mild and peaceful summer's day abruptly shattered by the appearance of a truck with a pig's soft pink snout poking out of the slats. The pleasantness of the day juxtaposed with the suffering of a being whose first breath of fresh air comes as a consequence of them eventually being taken to a gas chamber, where soon something else will be filling their lungs.

I now understand the machinations behind this systemic, systematic and relentless exploitation. A well-oiled system in which each part is tuned to a level of optimisation and efficiency that allows the cogs to keep on turning day after day, minute after minute, second after second. Not a single pause.

I now see through the adverts and marketing tricks of an industry that never stops working to obfuscate, hide and distract. The pictures and videos promoting happy animals and the labels that seek to reassure us that the body part wrapped in plastic came from an animal who was slaughtered and exploited with compassion and kindness.

Throughout this book, I have gone through the practical and behavioural challenges that are associated with veganism. However, for many vegans, the hardest part of being vegan is not about getting enough vitamin B12, finding tasty food or knowing which toiletries to buy. It's not even necessarily anything related to the practical aspects of going and staying vegan at all.

In all of the conversations I've had with other vegans throughout the years, the one challenge that has come up more than any other – which is also the one that I relate to the most – is living in a world where the dominant paradigm is the very thing that you are taking a stand against. In other words, being vegan in a non-vegan world.

Ignorance is bliss

For some of you, this might not be so much of a challenge. You might go vegan and find yourself accepting of the world around you and emotionally resilient to the reminders of what is happening to animals and the planet. You might have really supportive friends and family who are sincere and generous when it comes to you going vegan, making the process a breeze for you. It might even be the case that you are going vegan because you already have vegan friends, so you have an element of support and guidance from the outset.

For others, the disconnect between your values and what is actually happening to animals in the world might not be so easy to look past. Perhaps you once saw some footage from a farm or a slaughterhouse and you were reminded of it because of a meat aisle that you walked past when you were in a supermarket. Perhaps you saw an advert on the TV that was singing the praises of a welfare scheme or particular industry and you found yourself overcome with disappointment at just how misleading the messaging around animal farming is.

Sometimes when I'm out and about I'll see a poster advertising a food product like a burger, and my first reaction is to think that it's just a plant-based burger – then I remember that's not actually the case. Little moments like this can catch me off guard and remind me of what is happening to animals.

One thing you realise when you stop eating animal products is just how ubiquitous they are and how relentlessly they are marketed and advertised. They are visible everywhere all the time. Plus, the promotion of animal products is always framed in similar ways. It's always about how tasty they are and about how great the welfare standards and farming are. While these angles obviously make sense from a marketing perspective, it's so frustrating to have these narratives consistently shoved down our throats.

As a result, even simple things like going to a supermarket, going for a meal in a restaurant, watching TV or walking down the road include constant reminders of what is happening to animals and the scale of the problem at hand. All of a sudden, these everyday occurrences have a different aspect to them that we weren't used to before.

Going vegan can really show just how ignorant we once were and others still are to the issues that exist. Being ignorant is not in and of itself a criticism, though. There are lots of things that each of us does not know. However, in the case of veganism, what is notable is not just the scale of ignorance around the issues of animal exploitation, but also how this lack of awareness is not necessarily the fault of those who are unaware. This is prescribed ignorance, nurtured and fostered by extremely influential industries that can dominate messaging and advertising in such a way as to maintain a broad lack of unawareness in the people who support these industries through their purchases.

In the case of what we do to animals, this ignorance is predicated on the lie that animal farming is not an ethical, environmental or social-health issue. This is precisely why it's vital to challenge these industries by becoming more aware and changing our behaviour as a result. Even if the reality of the truth can at times be harder than the comfort of the lie, it is by acknowledging what needs to be changed that we can work towards creating a world where we don't need to hide behind a falsehood in order to feel comfortable.

The hardest pill to swallow

Advertising and marketing aren't necessarily the most challenging or jarring things that we have to deal with once we become vegan. It is one thing being vegan in a world where you are constantly reminded of what's happening to animals – it's another thing entirely when it is the people you love the most who are contributing to the persecution of animals.

In previous chapters, I outlined how to talk to friends and family about going vegan. I've also discussed dating and living with non-vegan partners. However, beyond the practical and conversational aspects, the other element of having non-vegan loved ones is the emotional toll that can arise as a consequence of seeing the people you love the most engaging in the thing that you are taking a stand against.

Perhaps you're having a lovely day with your family and then when it comes to dinnertime you catch a glimpse of a family member tucking in to a piece of meat. This makes you think about the animal they're eating and your mind is cast back to the video you saw of an animal struggling in a slaughterhouse. Maybe you're home for Christmas and you're having a nice day, but then there are dead animals on the table while everyone is pulling crackers, wearing party hats, laughing and having a good time.

It's these moments that can be the hardest part of being vegan – seeing a family member eating a piece of bacon or a ham sandwich and having to come to terms with the fact that our loved ones are paying to cause suffering. The gas chambers are not being controlled by someone evil, but as a result of the choices of the people who we love the most. We know that these are not cruel or bad people. In fact, they're the nicest, most compassionate and caring people we know. They're loving, considerate, empathetic *and* they pay for animals to be mutilated, exploited and slaughtered. That 'and' is so important, because it reveals how two different things can be true at once. Sadly, it's not a vegan multivitamin that's the hardest pill to swallow.

It's not even that we necessarily feel badly towards them. We might be disappointed and upset, but we still love and care about them. The severity of the discomfort is increased precisely because we are witnessing an apparent contradiction. People we feel strong affection, admiration and compassion for are eating the product of a system that we view as being inherently bad and therefore the antithesis of the person eating it.

This can put us in a tricky situation. We don't want to not see our loved ones, and we don't want to cause problems by having arguments. At the same time, not saying anything and acting like there is no problem can feel like a form of complicity that can make us feel guilty. We find ourselves walking a tightrope, whereby we are trying to balance as best we can while navigating this complex and at times emotionally challenging situation.

It's no wonder that being vegan in a non-vegan world can be so difficult. What, then, can we do about it?

The power of acceptance

If it is the case that you find yourself struggling with any of these issues, it is important to acknowledge them and find ways to deal with them. One of the most important things you can do is find a sense of acceptance. The world doesn't change overnight, and the important thing is that you have altered your behaviour to help be a part of that change. Beyond that, there is a limit to what you can do.

The idea of radical acceptance is a prominent one in psychology and therapy, and it consists of making a conscious effort to acknowledge how you feel and what is causing those feelings. Suffering can arise as a consequence of refusing to accept things that you don't have direct control over, so radical acceptance is the practice of finding a sense of liberation by accepting the reality of what is front of you, even if it is not what you would ideally like to be true.

Acceptance does not mean that you condone or approve of the thing that is troubling you – in this case, the abuse of animals. It instead means that you allow yourself to feel difficult emotions, but do so in a way that allows you to find a sense of space and objectivity around them. It is a common idea found within the philosophy of Stoicism, which encourages you to accept what you cannot control and focus on what you can.

The problem is, if you allow yourself to feel burdened and weighed down by a reality that you don't have the ability to change on your own, this can lead to you losing a sense of determination and conviction around your own choices. This can then morph into a sense of hopelessness and futility, which ultimately might impact your motivation to stay vegan. If your life is consumed by things you cannot change, and the one thing you can change is whether or not you are vegan, then you may come to the decision – albeit subconsciously – that the only way to alleviate your discomfort is to stop being vegan.

I've met people who used to be vegan who were so disheartened by what was going on and the lack of progress they felt was being made that it got to the point that they just couldn't see the value in staying vegan. Clearly this is not a helpful attitude or mindset to have, especially as the importance of us being vegan doesn't alter even if others are not changing as soon we'd like them to.

If we can instead accept the reality of what exists around us, this means that rather than viewing veganism as the source of our discomfort, we can view our choice to be vegan as the thing we have influence over. In other words, we can find comfort in our veganism, as it represents us living by our principles and values, and taking ownership of what it is that we can control.

If we get to a point where we're tired of feeling upset at our partner eating animal products, or we find ourselves wishing that we didn't have to justify our veganism at work or at a family gathering, it is understandable that we might then rationalise to ourselves that being vegan is the problem, and if we just stopped being vegan, everything would be fine. However, it is not the veganism that is the problem – it's the world around it.

While some people might decide no longer being vegan is the way to deal with any negative feelings, others sometimes decide to shut themselves off. They stop interacting with people who aren't vegan, or only do so when they are advocating for veganism, meaning the interactions can often be demoralising and further perpetuate their sense of isolation and disconnection. This is not the long-term solution either. Both of these options are examples of us attempting to externalise the issue by placing the source of our negative feelings outside of ourselves. However, while it might be the world around us that creates these feelings within us, we are ultimately the ones who can dictate how we process and respond to those feelings.

This is one of the core principles within forms of therapy such as cognitive behavioural therapy and dialectical behaviour therapy. It is also one of the overarching benefits of practising mindfulness. While suppressing our feelings, hiding from them or betraying our principles can offer a tempting short-term gain, it is not necessarily the case that those will help us in the long run.

There's a butcher's shop that I pass by fairly frequently on a very pleasant road with coffee shops, independent restaurants and clothing boutiques. On this street, it's very common to see a wide range of incredibly cute and happy dogs wagging their tails as they merrily enjoy being taken out for a walk. The road has a friendly hustle and bustle, generated by groups of friends relaxing and enjoying their days.

The butcher's shop on this pleasant road has a large window through which the owners display pieces of flesh from the assortment of dismembered animals they sell. This display includes all the usual cuts you'd expect from a butcher. However, sometimes I walk past and there will be a collection of ducks hanging by their necks, their lifeless feet dangling in the air, their bodies still intact and their heads pressed up against each other. On other occasions, they display the heads of pigs, their faces looking out at the road as people walk past with their speciality coffee in one hand and the lead that is attached to their very happy dog in the other. It is often the shock that catches me out – the brutality of the beheaded animal on display, their face providing a macabre visual representation of the all-encompassing nature of our domination over them. I then find myself grappling with the juxtaposition between the severed head and the overall geniality of the street the head looks out upon.

Sometimes these moments make me angry; sometimes they make me very sad. Sometimes I find myself ruminating on them for a considerable amount of time afterwards, rationalising to myself that everyone involved is awful – the owners are terrible people, and the consumers are beyond the pale. But, again, this is the easy thing to do. It's far simpler just to imagine that everyone involved in this butcher's shop is a terrible person and completely immoral. It allows me to neatly compartmentalise the problem and to create a binary of good and bad. However, it is not as straightforward as this.

While it's simpler to think badly of everyone involved in the existence of the butcher's shop, that overlooks the complexity of the situation and my own previous participation. How many butcher's shops did I walk past before I was vegan? How many butcher's shops did I eat meat from? How many severed heads were in the windows that went unnoticed?

I've bought ducks and I've bought meat from wild animals from butchers. I've bought meat from farmed animals, animals killed in gas chambers, animals who had their reproductive systems exploited, their babies taken from them and their lives filled with suffering. While I now classify all of these things as being bad, was I bad person when I bought them?

This question touches on one of the most vital and fundamental aspects of this discussion. It's really important that we decouple the problem from the people. Good people can do bad things. We are all a testament to that fact, as is the wider world around us.

This is especially the case when it comes to veganism, because consuming animal products is legally allowed, socially permissible, carried out by the majority of people and heavily advertised to us and pushed on us. None of these things mean that it is ethically acceptable as a result, but they provide essential context that explains why it is not as simple as viewing people as bad because they engage with industries that do bad things. Failing to understand this not only does a disservice to those people, but it can create a disconnection between ourselves and the people we love, and it can lead to a wider feeling of misanthropy.

Perspective and balance are so vital when it comes to being vegan. We can rightfully condemn the action of animal exploitation while at the same time understanding how such a system continues to be supported by people who are not evil or bad for doing so. In essence, to overcome the challenges that can arise from being vegan in a non-vegan world, we need to develop a level of emotional resilience and understanding.

Finding balance and perspective

While understanding the importance of balance and perspective can help immeasurably when it comes to dealing with the complexity of some of the feelings and emotions that can arise from being vegan, sometimes something will happen that will break its way through and impact you nonetheless. This could be something you see or something someone says to you.

I referenced behavioural therapy techniques as important tools by which we can gain a sense of emotional control, and such techniques are extremely valuable in these situations too. Let's say a work colleague has made some undermining comments to you, or maybe you've just walked past a butcher's shop and seen a decapitated pig's head displayed in the window. You might find yourself overcome with anger, sadness, guilt or shame.

If you find yourself in a situation like this, take a moment to pause and take a few deep breaths. From this point you can observe what your thoughts and feelings are and reflect on what has caused you to feel that way. Noticing your thoughts and feelings helps you find some space from them, which can reduce their severity and help you think more logically and rationally. From that position, it's then important to pull back and gain a sense of perspective. Is there a way that you can rationalise the situation and see it in context? For example, while unfair and not respectful, are your work colleague's comments more of a reflection of their behaviour and mindset than they are about you or your choice to be vegan? What led to them making those comments? Were they being defensive or grappling with their own cognitive dissonance?

In the example of the butcher's shop, when I feel shocked and sad, I try to reflect on that by adding the perspective that I can get from thinking it through in the ways I described earlier. I think about my actions before I was vegan, and I challenge the initial assumption that other people either don't care or are bad people.

Another really effective tool for reflection is to imagine that you are comforting a friend who is in the same situation you are in. For example, a vegan friend is really upset because they were mocked by a family member, or because they had an argument with a loved one. What would you say to them? This exercise is useful because we tend to be less critical, negative and judgemental when comforting our friends and loved ones. In such a scenario, we would most likely validate their experience and express empathy for why they feel the way they do, and then from that point we would seek to reassure them by providing more context and looking at the bigger picture. Viewing the situation from the perspective of a friend is especially important when it comes to situations where you might feel critical of yourself.

Once you've gained some helpful perspective, the next step is to try to find the best resolution to the situation. In some cases, this might be taking your mind off what has happened; for example, going for a walk, spending some time with a companion animal, watching videos of rescued animals in sanctuaries, making a cup of tea, listening to music or whatever it might be to help you move forward.

If you've had an argument, the best resolution could be to let the dust settle and then clear the air by trying to have a respectful conversation when the tension has dissipated. In the meantime, you can reflect on what went wrong, why the situation escalated and what you can do to make sure that it doesn't happen again.

When it comes to things outside of your control, the best resolution might be coming to terms with the reality of the situation. You could do this by accepting that this is how things are for the time being, and then reframe your mindset to be more positive by embracing the fact that you can feel proud of yourself for not being a part of that system.

In cognitive behavioural therapy, this practice is called STOPP:

S – Stop and pause
T – Take some deep breaths
O – Observe your thoughts and feelings
P – Pull back and gain some perspective
P – Proceed and move forward with the best resolution

Using this acronym can be a really helpful way of remembering the different steps. And even just saying STOPP can help you in a difficult situation by punctuating the moment and allowing you to create a sense of objectivity and control over your feelings and emotions.

Never miss an opportunity to feel positive

As well as having practices and techniques that can help you in the moment, you also want to be working towards a long-term sense of wellbeing. One really helpful way of doing this is to look out for things that are positive and remind yourself of them frequently. If you only view veganism through the lens of it being a way to combat a complex global problem, you can run the risk of viewing success through that lens as well and missing out on the more localised, single-issue or smaller positive actions and outcomes that are all around us.

If the bar for what you deem positive or a success story is set too high, you can fall into the trap of consistently feeling negative or like there is no change happening. But this isn't true. While system change is a long process that can feel arduous and unobtainable at times, that doesn't mean there are not reasons to feel optimistic along the way.

For example, there are stories being reported all the time about how greyhound racing or bullfighting is being banned in different places, how marine protected areas are being expanded and certain types of fishing prohibited, how aquariums are closing their doors or ending their captive breeding programmes, and how sales of meat are in decline in certain countries, to name but a few. And every day that you live by your vegan principles is a success and something you should feel positive about.

Even something like cell-cultured meat, which has the capacity to create a positive impact around the world, won't change things overnight – there will be lots of incremental changes over a period of time. However, if you view each and every one of these incremental changes as not being enough, then you are pinning your positive outlook on something that will not happen in the way you necessarily want it to. Instead, you should view every step on that journey as a success and something to feel positive about.

We sometimes do this with our own personal pursuits of happiness and success. We might think, *Once X happens, then I'll be happy*, or, *If I was just able to do Y, then I would feel like I had achieved something.* Measuring our ability to feel happy or positive via a condition that might not be met, or might not occur in the way that we thought it would, means that we are placing barriers in front of ourselves that can impact our ability to feel positive, happy or successful.

In the case of veganism, you might also feel guilty if you sometimes feel positive about things. Perhaps you had a productive conversation, read an encouraging piece of news or cooked a delicious plant-based meal for your friends, and you feel positive and happy about it. You might then have a tendency to undermine that emotion by thinking about what's still happening to animals and subsequently feel ashamed that you allowed yourself to feel positive or happy about something while all of the problems in the world continue. However, punishing yourself or being consumed with unwarranted guilt isn't going to help you in the long term – if anything, it will just reinforce a negative mindset that might even impact whether you stay vegan in the future or not. Plus, not allowing yourself to feel positive or to celebrate successes, no matter how small, doesn't bring about change any quicker. If you forbid yourself from feeling proud or happy for positively representing veganism, that doesn't suddenly alleviate the suffering and exploitation the animals are facing.

While there are plenty of negative things happening to animals, there are positive strides being made too, and we can and should celebrate these, no matter how small they may seem. So, even though veganism views the issue of animal exploitation as a whole, we can still derive positivity from some of the more specific changes that are happening around us. Large change tends to occur because of a collection of smaller changes happening in pursuit of that wider goal. As such, every positive story, conversation and event is worth celebrating and feeling good about. If you're interested in keeping up to date with positive vegan news, I have a newsletter where I share regular roundups of all the inspiring things that have been happening in the world of veganism. You can sign up to my newsletter by going to my website, which is earthlinged.org.

Our identities beyond veganism

It's also important that you make time for your hobbies, interests and other passions. While veganism might become a big part of who you are, it's not your whole identity, and being vegan isn't the only thing that defines you. I know from my personal experience, as well as from the experiences of other vegans I know, that we can sometimes become so passionate about being vegan that we forget to nurture other areas of our lives.

It is vital to spend time away from thinking about the issues and injustices that we see. Veganism and animal exploitation are no different. If you spend all of your time thinking, talking and consuming content about the ethical, social and environmental issues relating to the consumption of animals, then it will begin to weigh heavy on your mind and could very easily lead to you feeling isolated, frustrated and negative.

Earlier, when I discussed the idea of trying to come to terms with uncomfortable things that are out of your control, I mentioned that one way of helping with that is to try and positively influence others. For example, if you're feeling upset about the state of the world, you can channel that emotion and use it as fuel to try and do something positive about it.

For most advocates, myself included, it is these feelings that form the driving force behind our advocacy. What it means to be an advocate is entirely up to you though. For some people, it might mean joining events, marches and community-building activism. For others, being an advocate might mean bringing vegan food in to work for people to try, or cooking vegan food for your non-vegan friends and family.

There is no one-size-fits-all approach to being an advocate, and what you find most fulfilling or enjoyable will depend on who you are and what you find most valuable. If you can combine a form of advocacy with a hobby or passion, then that can also be really rewarding. However, if you find that a certain form of advocacy doesn't resonate with you, or you try something and it doesn't have a positive impact in the way that you hoped, re-evaluating and trying something different is also absolutely fine.

The point about making time to nurture the other aspects of our lives and identities is even more important if you do decide to become more involved in vegan advocacy work, whatever it may be. Advocating for veganism can be a really rewarding and positive experience, but you need time away from it too. For example, if your weekdays are spent at work with colleagues who tease you frequently, and then on an evening you're consuming vegan content or engaging with people online about veganism, and then at the weekend you go to an event to promote veganism – it's clear that a significant amount of your time and energy is going to be taken up by being absorbed in the world of veganism.

Sadly, and this doesn't just apply to vegan advocacy, I have known people who became so invested in their activism that they burned out. Obviously, this is of no help to anyone, including those who you were advocating on behalf of. It can be easy to feel guilty if you don't think you are doing everything you can, but you have to make time for other aspects of your life too.

This is one of the things that if I could turn back time to when I first went vegan, I would make sure I did differently. I jumped right in with advocating for veganism, and it's not that I regret doing so – far from it – it's that I wish that I had given myself more time to engage in my other interests too. When I made that adjustment, not only did I feel like my advocacy actually became more effective, but I felt like my life and identity became more balanced too.

In essence, if you like movies, gigs, nights out, reading, hiking, going out for meals, playing video games or whatever else you enjoy doing, then make sure that you're still nurturing that side of who you are. In the case of activities where you might find yourself uncomfortably reminded of what is happening to animals, it is again important to find the space to acknowledge your feelings, implement those techniques I mentioned previously and practise acceptance – not because you condone the situation, but because it can help you deal with the negative feelings that might arise.

Dismissing the noise

Another aspect of living vegan in a non-vegan world is dealing with the misinformation and disinformation around veganism and plant-based diets. You can go on social media and hear all kinds of stories about how vegetables are toxic, almonds are leaching your body of nutrients, seed oils are the biggest public-health threat facing humanity and that we should be eating more meat. However, it's important to dismiss the noise and critically evaluate the quality of evidence and information that we are receiving. This is why it's important to make sure to follow the advice of trusted and reliable sources. The opinions, views and anecdotes of people online don't change the evidence. If a video on social media declares that a plant-based diet isn't healthy, that shouldn't carry more weight in our minds than the position of the British Dietetic Association or the NHS.

The same is true of environmental claims. In recent years, it has become exceptionally common for people to claim that animal farming isn't as bad as we're told and that cattle grazing in particular is sustainable. Yet, over the same period of time, more and more high-quality scientific research has been published that disputes these claims.

Environmental organisations and health authorities decide their positions based on an evaluation of the totality of evidence available. It is incredibly frustrating, therefore, when these claims are disregarded because of a cherry-picked study or because of an ideological position. A prime example of this was Elon Musk declaring on Joe Rogan's podcast that animal farming has 'zero' impact on global warming. Common sense alone should tell you this is wrong, but the fact that reports about the environmental impact of animal farming come from the largest and most comprehensive studies that adhere to the highest standards of scientific evidence should provide all the proof anyone should need. The fact that Musk and Rogan would make and discuss such bogus claims without providing any evidence whatsoever points to either a significant level of cognitive dissonance or an attempt to spread disinformation deliberately. Either way, their desire to deny or obfuscate the truth leads to a delegitimisation of actual evidence and spreads doubt about the impact of meat, dairy and eggs in the minds of the people who are listening.

The tactic of spreading doubt is a very common tool used by industries under threat to disrupt the information landscape and make the public question the legitimacy of the evidence they are receiving. It is a tactic that has been used by the tobacco, fossil fuel and animal agriculture industries. By working with pseudoscientists and PR firms, they can create campaigns of disinformation that warp people's opinions and views about important issues. In the case of veganism, we see this regularly with attacks on plant-based alternatives and attempts to redeem the image of red meat in particular.

In January 2019, a groundbreaking study was published called the EAT-*Lancet* report[1] that analysed how to feed a growing population without causing catastrophic climate breakdown. It was published in one of the most highly respected scientific journals in the world and was a collaborative project with an international team of researchers. One of its recommendations was for a global reduction in red-meat consumption. Perhaps unsurprisingly, leaked minutes from a meeting of the Animal Agriculture Alliance, a meat, dairy and egg coalition group with representatives and members from the largest animal agriculture companies in the world, showed that the alliance was concerned about the report over a month before it was published.[2]

In response to the report, a PR firm called Red Flag, which itself had previously worked with the meat and dairy sector, represented the Animal Agriculture Alliance in a campaign which attempted to discredit the EAT-*Lancet* report.[3] What followed was a global campaign that spread talking points that painted the researchers and paper as being hypocritical and radical. That sparked a backlash against the report from others.

In the weeks following its publication, hundreds of articles about the EAT-*Lancet* report included messaging and quotes from Red Flag, and thousands of critical posts were shared on Twitter (now X). The negative coverage quickly outnumbered neutral or positive stories. This led to the report being undermined in the minds of the public. However, the report remains hugely influential and groundbreaking within the scientific community, having been cited more than 9,000 times since its publication. It is also among the papers most often cited by governments and in policy briefs.

The bottom line is we might come across content that claims that a plant-based diet can't be healthy or that animal farming isn't bad for the environment, but the totality of evidence shows that both of these claims are incorrect. This is precisely why we should listen to our leading health and environmental organisations and ignore those who are either biased or ill-informed.

Acknowledging the absurdity

In 2025, an American hunter by the name of Sam Jones uploaded a video of herself picking up a baby wombat when she was in Australia and temporarily separating them from their mother for a social media video. This video sparked an enormous amount of criticism, especially in Australia, where the prime minister, Anthony Albanese, stated during a press conference that 'to take a baby wombat from its mother, and clearly causing distress from the mother, is just an outrage'. He then challenged the hunter to take a baby crocodile from their mother and see how she got on.

While Jones had clearly done something wrong, the outrage at a baby animal being forcibly taken from their mother was absurdly ironic. After all, the separation of families is an inherent part of animal exploitation. The most infamous example of this occurs in the dairy industry, where newborn calves are taken from their mothers shortly after being born. There is one significant difference though: Jones gave the baby wombat back to their mother, something that farmers don't do with the baby animals they steal. So, is it not also an outrage for a baby calf, piglet, lamb or other animal to be taken from their mother, causing distress to both the baby and the mother?

This story and others like it demonstrate the paradoxical nature of our relationship with animals. While this absurdity is not always so noticeable to non-vegans, it is one aspect of living in a non-vegan world that can certainly raise an eyebrow from us vegans. I am of course glad that some acts of harm are condemned, but I do sometimes find myself frozen with a sense of disbelief at just how contradictory and inconsistent our ethics and values towards animals really are.

It also becomes apparent just how meaningless some claims made about animal products are. It seems like everywhere you go, whether it's a butcher's shop, supermarket or restaurant, there is always a point made about how the meat is sustainable and ethical. On top of this, everywhere only seems to sell sustainably caught seafood. Before going vegan, you might accept this at face value, or at least allow yourself to believe it for peace of mind. However, when you go vegan, you realise just how frequently the message that the animal products we eat are all sustainable and ethical is pushed on us. It's no wonder consumers are so confused. If you were to trust all of this messaging, it would seem impossible to think anything other than that the animal products sold where you live are not part of the problem.

Not only that, it seems like all animal products come from local farms. This is such a common message that people assume that it means something valuable. However, environmental science shows us that local food doesn't mean sustainable food,[4] and from an ethical perspective, the distance the food has travelled doesn't change the morality of how it was produced. Even the biggest and most intensive farms are local to someone, and the immorality of those farms doesn't change based on our geographical relation to them.

Similarly, every fishmonger only sells fresh fish. What does this even mean? Advertising that the fish you serve isn't rotten would hardly be a glowing endorsement. Worse still, many places advertise that they serve local fish, which considering I live in London and the only local water is the River Thames is certainly cause for concern, as it is not known for being especially clean – although this applies to just about all rivers in the UK thanks to sewage companies and the animal farming industries, both of which pollute our rivers and streams with faeces. I am of course being slightly tongue-in-cheek – the fish sold in London are clearly not being sourced from the River Thames. However, the fact that seafood served in London can be called 'local' just shows what a farce these terms are.

But despite the absurdity, we are constantly having these labels and phrases thrust upon us. We're told not to worry because animal products are: fresh, local, sustainably sourced, sustainability caught, sustainably farmed, ethical, high-welfare, humanely raised, humanely slaughtered, outdoor-reared, outdoor-bred, RSPCA Assured, Red Tractor-approved, MSC-certified. Also, did I mention that they're free-range, outdoor-grazed, grass-fed, family-farmed, regeneratively farmed, traceable, organic and happy? The animals are always happy. And did I mention local?

One of the most absurd contradictions that becomes noticeable once you go vegan is just how secretive and censored animal farming is. We're told that our treatment of animals is ethical and humane, but if you share footage from a slaughterhouse on social media, it will be blocked, removed or censored. Weirdly enough, animal farming is so humane and ethical that you can't show it to people.

Moody pigs and unfriendly goats

As well as noticing the many absurdities and contradictions of animal exploitation and consumption, the flip side is that you might also notice that you gain a wider appreciation of animals more generally. By reframing our perception of animals and viewing them as individuals deserving of moral consideration, we are fostering a mentality that encourages us to view them more for who they are. The positive consequence can be that we find ourselves appreciating animals more than we used to.

I noticed this when I realised that I had become invested in the lives of two pigeons that I would always see through my window. The pigeons were a couple and would always sit in the same spots and hang out together. Whereas before I wouldn't have even realised that they were the same pigeons, I found myself fascinated by the fact that these two individuals were living this whole life together. They had their own schedule and habits, and while I was absorbed in my own world and living my life, around me they were living their own lives too.

For many people, the idea of caring about two pigeons would seem farcical and would be met with derision. Yet it can be oddly comforting to acknowledge the intricacies and scope of life and experience that exists all around us. We can sometimes become so wrapped up in our own lives, worries and anxieties, goals and pursuits, that we can become disconnected from the world around us.

One of the reasons why we love having pets so much is that they can bring us joy and fulfilment. After all, it's not only vegans who find it calming to watch a cat curled up on the sofa fast asleep. When we have animals in our lives, we develop a deeper and greater understanding of their personalities, and that nourishes and enriches us too. The fact that the animals we have in our homes are living their own lives means that we spend time pondering what they're thinking and feeling. This speaks to a desire for a greater understanding and appreciation.

I strongly believe that veganism can do something similar, but can expand the desire for understanding beyond just those animals who we might more conventionally find ourselves interested in. One time when I was in a park in London, a family was watching a squirrel eating, remarking on how cute they were. All of a sudden, they saw a rat next to the squirrel, who also was just sat there eating. However, they referred to the rat as disgusting and unpleasant. The difference between a rat and squirrel is small to say the least. Both are rodents, albeit with different tails and different reputations. The truth is I would have probably felt something similar before I was vegan. In fact, there's a strong chance that as well as being repulsed by the rat, I would have simply felt indifferent to the squirrel.

In the same way that I find a cat asleep on the sofa both calming and cause for introspection, I now find myself experiencing something similar watching a pigeon couple sitting on a tree branch living their own lives. I feel especially grateful for this change in attitude.

Appreciating animals more doesn't just mean viewing them through rose-tinted glasses. I've met moody pigs, unfriendly goats, and chickens that are more than happy to peck you. However, I don't view this as a negative at all. We're so used to thinking of animals in abstract ways that remove any sense of personality from them that we often fall into the trap of perceiving them as being broadly the same. Animals have a variety of personalities, and while there are plenty of cute, friendly and gentle animals, there are plenty who are the opposite. There are some more intelligent than others, some more naughty than others, some more kind than others. None of these things change the fact that it's wrong to exploit them – if anything, the complexity and diversity of their experiences just further proves why it's wrong in the first place.

So, while being vegan in a non-vegan world can bring with it emotional challenges and discomfort, especially in the case of friends and family, it can also change our perspective on things in ways that can be enriching. This change might be subtle; after all, it could just seem like we are thinking about animals in a more considered way than we did previously. However, while seemingly subtle, this change might speak to a deeper and more profound shift in perspective than we initially realise.

CONCLUSION

The football manager Bill Shankly once said: 'Football is a simple game made complicated.' In many ways, veganism is the same. At its core, it is simply about making choices to reduce the exploitation and harm of animals. It is as straightforward as picking up tofu in a supermarket instead of chicken, and opting for one of the many brands of plant milk over cows' milk. However, while it may be simple in principle, there are a number of social, cultural and psychological barriers that can stand in the way of us becoming and staying vegan and that therefore need to be overcome.

If we overlook these challenges, we run the risk of not being prepared and ultimately failing to reach our goal. This is why understanding and acknowledging the barriers that can get in the way is of huge importance. Through doing so, we can put strategies in place to overcome them and learn from our mistakes and experiences along the way.

Being prepared is key to so many things in life – veganism is no different. I hope that after reading this book you have more awareness of what to look out for and what the challenges can be, and, most importantly, you now have the knowledge of how to deal with them if or when they arise.

However, in the same way that Bill Shankly's quote about football pokes fun at the overanalysing that can go into the sport, the change to veganism can also be viewed in such a way as to burden it with an unnecessary sense of hardship and difficulty. This can make veganism seem daunting and unobtainable in the eyes of many. With that in mind, I also hope that I have demystified the process of going vegan and that it now seems less complicated and more achievable than it did before.

Enrichment through change

While some people view veganism as restrictive, I believe it is less about limiting what we choose to eat and more about expanding what we choose to acknowledge and act upon. It is about turning our backs on the restrictive nature of wilful ignorance and understanding the reality of what is happening to animals, even if doing so doesn't always reveal something comfortable or pleasant. It is by doing this that we can then act according to our principles and in alignment with the type of person we aspire to be.

This is why going vegan is one of the most important and rewarding decisions that you can make. First, because it addresses the harm associated with our food, clothing, toiletries and entertainment, and second, because it goes beyond just dealing with the tangible symptoms of the problem. Going vegan is about challenging cultural and social norms, re-evaluating our own behaviours and mindsets, championing a change in how we treat our planet and opposing the dominant ethical paradigm of animal exploitation. Veganism also encourages us to find out more about ourselves, what we can accomplish and what our principles and values are. It is therefore both personally fulfilling and rewarding, while also being extremely consequential.

The common perception of veganism is that it is to deprive yourself of something. Even those who view veganism in a more favourable light often perceive it as a noble cause that comes at the cost of an individual's own personal happiness.

But this doesn't need to be the case. While it can be inconvenient at times, and while we can feel saddened by what is happening to animals or frustrated by some of the conversations we might have with others, being vegan doesn't have to be all doom and gloom. It can also be incredibly enjoyable: it can lead to discovering new foods, flavours and ingredients; becoming a more confident and capable cook; having a greater understanding of how to be healthy; developing more confidence in ourselves and what we can achieve; and having a more enriching perspective towards animals.

Go for it

It is likely that you will have come across parts of this book that aren't entirely relevant to your life right now; however, that may well change in the future. Perhaps you will begin dating a non-vegan, move in with some non-vegan friends or think about getting a companion animal. Even if these things happen years from now, this book will always be here for you when you need it.

Also, if you slip up, make mistakes or find yourself back on page 1 again, what is important is not the fact that you slipped up, but that you have decided to go again. Life isn't about being perfect or never making a mistake; it's about the progress we make and the way we develop and change over time. Like I mentioned right at the beginning, this book is your non-judgemental companion, and it will remain that way if you find yourself eating a non-vegan pizza or even if you fall off the vegan wagon completely. However, every day that we live by our principles and therefore contribute to creating a better world is a day that we can be proud of ourselves.

All of this brings me to my final piece of advice. You've got to the end of the book and now is your chance to put into practice everything that has been covered on the pages preceding this one. I know what it's like to reach the point where you are on the precipice of making the change and going vegan. It can feel daunting and intimidating, and you can find yourself pushing back the day you plan to make the change; however, many vegans once found themselves in that same situation. So don't worry if this is the way that you feel, or if you still have a sense of apprehension – committing to going vegan is one of the hardest parts of the change itself.

However, becoming vegan is also exciting, empowering and rewarding. It presents us with an opportunity to grow, learn and discover more about ourselves – and, importantly, in our own lives and for the lives of animals and for the health of our planet, there is also so much to be gained from going vegan. So be kind to yourself, take it one step at a time, have fun and remember, you've got this.

RESOURCES

Listed below are a selection of useful resources that I have found to be incredibly helpful during my time as a vegan. I have split them into different categories to make them easier to navigate.

At the very end is a meal planner template that you can copy and use to plan out what delicious plant-based meals you are going to be eating each day – this can be especially useful in the early days before eating a vegan diet has become second nature to you. If you're looking for inspiration, you can refer back to the breakfast, lunch and dinner ideas that I listed in Chapter 3. Alternatively, I have also included a list of websites that have a great selection of plant-based recipes available on them.

General Help and Guidance
Veganuary:
https://www.veganuary.com

The Vegan Society:
https://www.vegansociety.com

Ethics
Animal Equality:
https://animalequality.org.uk

Animal Aid:
https://www.animalaid.org.uk

Viva!:
https://viva.org.uk/

Animal Justice Project:
https://www.animaljusticeproject.com/

Dominion (documentary):
https://www.dominionmovement.com/watch

Health

British Dietetic Association:
https://www.bda.uk.com/resource/vegetarian-vegan-plant-based-diet.html
https://www.bda.uk.com/resource/plant-based-eating-for-beginners.html

NHS:
https://www.nhs.uk/live-well/eat-well/how-to-eat-a-balanced-diet/the-vegan-diet

Plant-Based Health Professionals:
https://plantbasedhealthprofessionals.com

The Vegan Society:
https://www.vegansociety.com/resources/nutrition-and-health

Nutrition Facts:
https://nutritionfacts.org

Vegan Parenting

The Vegan Society:
https://www.vegansociety.com/resources/nutrition-and-health/life-stages

RESOURCES

NHS:
https://www.nhs.uk/pregnancy/keeping-well/vegetarian-or-vegan-and-pregnant

Plant-Based Health Professionals:
https://plantbasedhealthprofessionals.com/factsheets-for-pregnancy-children

Social Media:
You can find vegan parenting groups on social media platforms such as Facebook. If you're looking to connect with other vegan parents or find out more about raising your children vegan, these groups can be really helpful.

Recipes

The following list of recipe resources is far from exhaustive; however, all these resources have a great selection of different plant-based meals and are fantastic sources of inspiration if you are searching for new meals to try. If you are looking for a recipe for a particular dish, then one of the easiest ways to find it is to just search for it on the internet. For example, you can search for 'vegan lasagna recipe' or 'creamy vegan korma recipe', and you will find lots of different options that you can then choose from.

Deliciously Ella:
https://www.deliciouslyella.com

BOSH!:
https://www.bosh.tv/

Rainbow Plant Life:
https://rainbowplantlife.com

BBC Good Food:
https://www.bbcgoodfood.com

Epicurious:
https://www.epicurious.com

Where to Buy Plant-Based Ingredients

Thankfully, the staples of a plant-based diet can be found almost everywhere; however, some plant-based foods are not always as easy to find. Most major supermarket chains offer a selection of plant-based alternatives, although the amount can vary depending on the supermarket and the size of the store. Ordering online for a home delivery is often the best way of accessing the full range of products that the supermarkets sell, and it can also be helpful to check different supermarkets, as they often stock different products and brands.

Sometimes plant-based recipes can call for niche ingredients that are not available from many supermarkets; for example, I reference an ingredient called kala namak (or black salt). These ingredients can often be found in health food stores instead, such as Holland & Barrett or independent organic stores. Alternatively, they can usually be found easily online.

Alcohol
Barnivore:
https://www.barnivore.com/

Travelling
Happy Cow:
https://www.happycow.net

Abillion:
https://www.abillion.com

Clothing
You can find clothes suitable for vegans in most high-street stores, although there can still be ethical concerns

around these brands, even if the items are suitable for vegans. If you are looking for something in particular, then searching online is a really easy way of finding what the options are; for example, if you're looking for a style of footwear, a type of coat or an item that uses organic or recycled materials.

Collective Fashion Justice:
https://www.collectivefashionjustice.org

Good On You:
https://goodonyou.eco

Cosmetics and Toiletries
Leaping Bunny Program (includes a list of all certified brands): https://www.leapingbunny.org

Boots
https://www.boots.com

Lush
https://www.lush.com

Superdrug
https://www.superdrug.com

Holland & Barrett
https://www.hollandandbarrett.com

Sephora
https://www.sephora.co.uk

Cult Beauty
https://www.cultbeauty.co.uk

Household Cleaning Products
Leaping Bunny Program (includes a list of all certified brands): https://www.leapingbunny.org

Astonish
https://astonish.co.uk

Ecover
https://uk.ecover.com

Method
https://methodproducts.co.uk

Waitrose own brand

Sainsbury's own brand

Marks & Spencer own brand

Asda own brand

Vegan News
My newsletter, which you can subscribe to by visiting:
https://earthlinged.org

Sentient Media:
https://sentientmedia.org

Plant Based News:
https://plantbasednews.org

Animal Adoption
Again, the list below is not exhaustive, and there are many smaller animal rescues and adoption centres that you can re-home animals from. There's also a strong chance that there will be local animal rescue organisations near where you live that you can support, and they might also be best equipped to offer you any post-rescue help and guidance if you choose to adopt through them.

RSPCA:
https://www.rspca.org.uk/findapet

RESOURCES

Blue Cross:
https://www.bluecross.org.uk

Battersea Dogs and Cats Home:
https://www.battersea.org.uk

Cats Protection:
https://www.cats.org.uk

Dogs Trust:
https://www.dogstrust.org.uk

Rabbit Welfare Association & Fund:
https://rabbitwelfare.co.uk/rehoming-rabbits/

WEEKLY MEAL PLANNER

WEEK _____

	BREAKFAST	LUNCH	DINNER	SNACKS
MON				
TUE				
WED				
THU				
FRI				
SAT				
SUN				

NOTES

CHAPTER 1: WHY VEGAN?

1. Our World in Data, 'Land animals slaughtered for meat, World, 1961 to 2023': https://ourworldindata.org/grapher/land-animals-slaughtered-for-meat
2. Mood, A. and Brooke, P., 'Estimating global numbers of fishes caught from the wild annually from 2000 to 2009', *Animal Welfare* 33 (2024), p. e6: https://doi.org/10.1017/awf.2024.7.
3. Antimicrobial Resistance Collaborators, 'Global burden of bacterial antimicrobial resistance in 2019: a systematic analysis', *The Lancet* 399(10325) (2022): https://doi.org/10.1016/S0140-6736(21)02724-0
4. Ritchie, H. and Spooner, F., 'Large amounts of antibiotics are used in livestock, but several countries have shown this doesn't have to be the case', Our World in Data (9 December 2024): https://ourworldindata.org/antibiotics-livestock
5. Save Our Antibiotics, *Case Study of a Health Crisis: How Human Health Is Under Threat from Over-Use of Antibiotics in Intensive Livestock Farming* (2011): https://www.saveourantibiotics.org/media/1491/case-study-of-a-health-crisis.pdf
6. Mulchandani, R., Wang, Y., Gilbert, M. and Van Boeckel, T.P., 'Global trends in antimicrobial use in food-producing animals: 2020 to 2030', *PLOS Global Public Health* 3(2) (2023): https://doi.org/10.1371/journal.pgph.0001305
7. Cui, M., Shen, B., Fu, Z.F. and Chen, H., 'Animal diseases and human future', *Animal Diseases* 2(1) (2022): https://animaldiseases.biomedcentral.com/articles/10.1186/s44149-022-00041-z
8. United Nations Environment Programme and International Livestock Research Institute, *Preventing the Next Pandemic: Zoonotic Diseases and How to Break the Chain of Transmission* (2020): https://unsdg.un.org/sites/default/files/2020-07/UNEP-Preventing-the-next-pandemic.pdf

9. Aune, D., 'Meat consumption and type 2 diabetes', *The Lancet Diabetes and Endocrinology* 12(9) (2024): https://doi.org/10.1016/S2213-8587(24)00198-0
10. Qian, F., Liu, G., Hu, F.B., Bhupathiraju, S.N. and Sun, Q., 'Association between plant-based dietary patterns and risk of type 2 diabetes: a systematic review and meta-analysis', *JAMA Internal Medicine* 179(10) (2019): https://doi.org/10.1001/jamainternmed.2019.2195
11. Papier, K., Knuppel, A., Syam, N., Jebb, S.A. and Key, T.J., 'Meat consumption and risk of ischemic heart disease: a systematic review and meta-analysis', *Critical Reviews in Food Science and Nutrition* 63(3) (2021): https://doi.org/10.1080/10408398.2021.1949575
12. Wang, Y., Liu, B., Han, H. et al., 'Associations between plant-based dietary patterns and risks of type 2 diabetes, cardiovascular disease, cancer, and mortality – a systematic review and meta-analysis', *Nutrition Journal* 22(1) (2023): https://doi.org/10.1186/s12937-023-00877-2
13. Di, Y., Ding, L., Gao, L. and Huang, H., 'Association of meat consumption with the risk of gastrointestinal cancers: a systematic review and meta-analysis', *BMC Cancer* 23(1) (2023): https://doi.org/10.1186/s12885-023-11218-1
14. Wang, Liu, Han, et al., op. cit.
15. World Health Organization, 'Cardiovascular diseases (CVDs)' (11 June 2021): https://www.who.int/news-room/fact-sheets/detail/cardiovascular-diseases-(cvds)
16. Cancer Research UK, 'Bowel cancer statistics': https://www.cancerresearchuk.org/health-professional/cancer-statistics/statistics-by-cancer-type/bowel-cancer
17. World Health Organization, 'Cancer': https://www.who.int/news-room/fact-sheets/detail/cancer
18. Capodici, A., Mocciaro, G., Gori, D., et al., 'Cardiovascular health and cancer risk associated with plant based diets: an umbrella review', *PLoS ONE* 19(5) (2024): https://doi.org/10.1371/journal.pone.0300711
19. Springmann, M., Godfray, H.C.J., Rayner, M. and Scarborough, P., 'Analysis and valuation of the health and climate change cobenefits of dietary change', *Proceedings of the National Academy of Sciences of the United States of America* 113(15) (2016): https://doi.org/10.1073/pnas.1523119113
20. Ritchie, H., Rosado, P. and Roser, M., 'Meat and dairy production', Our World in Data (August 2017; December 2023): https://ourworldindata.org/meat-production
21. Ritchie, H., 'How much of global greenhouse gas emissions come from food?', Our World in Data (18 March 2021): https://ourworldindata.org/greenhouse-gas-emissions-food

22. Ritchie, H., 'What share of global CO_2 emissions come from aviation?', Our World in Data (8 April 2024): https://ourworldindata.org/global-aviation-emissions
23. Clark, M.A., Domingo, N.G.G., Colgan, K., et al., 'Global food system emissions could preclude achieving the 1.5° and 2°C climate change targets', *Science* 370(6517) (2020): https://doi.org/10.1126/science.aba7357
24. United Nations Environment Programme, 'Global assessment: urgent steps must be taken to reduce methane emissions this decade' (6 May 2021): https://www.unep.org/news-and-stories/press-release/global-assessment-urgent-steps-must-be-taken-reduce-methane
25. Ritchie, H., Rosado, P. and Roser, M., 'Breakdown of carbon dioxide, methane and nitrous oxide emissions by sector', Our World in Data (June 2020; January 2024): https://ourworldindata.org/emissions-by-sector
26. Reisinger, A., Clark, H., Cowie, A.L., et al., 'How necessary and feasible are reductions of methane emissions from livestock to support stringent temperature goals?', *Philosophical Transactions of the Royal Society A: Mathematical, Physical and Engineering Sciences* 379(2210) (2021): https://doi.org/10.1098/rsta.2020.0452
27. Ritchie, Rosado and Roser, op. cit.
28. Ritchie, H., Rosado, P. and Roser, M., 'Greenhouse gas emissions', Our World in Data (June 2020; January 2024): https://ourworldindata.org/greenhouse-gas-emissions
29. Ritchie, H. and Rosado, M., 'Half of the world's habitable land is used for agriculture', Our World in Data (16 February 2024): https://ourworldindata.org/global-land-for-agriculture
30. Poore, J. and Nemecek, T., 'Reducing food's environmental impacts through producers and consumers', *Science* 360(6392) (2018): https://www.science.org/doi/10.1126/science.aaq0216
31. Benton, T.G., Bieg, C., Harwatt, H., Pudasaini, R. and Wellesley, L., *Food System Impacts on Biodiversity Loss: Three Levers for Food System Transformation in Support of Nature*, Chatham House (2021): https://www.chathamhouse.org/sites/default/files/2021-02/2021-02-03-food-system-biodiversity-loss-benton-et-al_0.pdf
32. Ritchie, H., 'Drivers of deforestation', Our World in Data (February 2021; May 2024): https://ourworldindata.org/drivers-of-deforestation
33. De Ruiter, H., Macdiarmid, J.I., Matthews, R.B., et al., 'Total global agricultural land footprint associated with UK food supply 1986–2011', *Global Environmental Change* 43 (2017): https://doi.org/10.1016/j.gloenvcha.2017.01.007
34. Harwatt, H. and Hayek, M.N., *Eating Away at Climate Change with Negative Emissions: Repurposing UK Agricultural Land to Meet Climate Goals*, Harvard Law School (2019): https://animal.law.harvard.edu/

wp-content/uploads/Eating-Away-at-Climate-Change-with-Negative-Emissions%E2%80%93%E2%80%93Harwatt-Hayek.pdf
35. Phillips, H., De Palma, A., Gonzalez, R.E., et al., *The Biodiversity Intactness Index – Country, Region and Global-Level Summaries for the Year 1970 to 2050 Under Various Scenarios*, Natural History Museum (2021): https://doi.org/10.5519/he1eqmg1
36. Poore and Nemecek, op. cit.
37. Gephart, J.A., Henriksson, P.J.G., Parker, R.W.R., et al., 'Environmental performance of blue foods', *Nature* 597 (2021): https://doi.org/10.1038/s41586-021-03889-2
38. United Nations Climate Action, 'The ocean – the world's greatest ally against climate change': https://www.un.org/en/climatechange/science/climate-issues/ocean
39. Ibid.
40. Mariani, G., Cheung, W.W.L., Lyet, A., et al., 'Let more big fish sink: fisheries prevent blue carbon sequestration – half in unprofitable areas', *Science Advances* 6(44) (2020): https://doi.org/10.1126/sciadv.abb4848
41. Ritchie, H. and Roser, M., 'Fish and overfishing', Our World in Data (October 2021; March 2024): https://ourworldindata.org/fish-and-overfishing
42. Scarborough, P., Clark, M., Cobiac, L., et al., 'Vegans, vegetarians, fish-eaters and meat-eaters in the UK show discrepant environmental impacts', *Nature Food* 4 (2023): https://doi.org/10.1038/s43016-023-00795-w

CHAPTER 2: A NEW NORMAL
1. Wise, P.M., Nattress, L., Flammer, L.J. and Beauchamp, G.K., 'Reduced dietary intake of simple sugars alters perceived sweet taste intensity but not perceived pleasantness', *American Journal of Clinical Nutrition* 103(1) (2016): https://doi.org/10.3945/ajcn.115.112300

CHAPTER 3: HOW TO NAVIGATE FOOD
1. Springmann, M., Clark, M.A., Rayner, M., Scarborough, P. and Webb, P., 'The global and regional costs of healthy and sustainable dietary patterns: a modelling study', *The Lancet Planetary Health* 5(11) (2021): https://doi.org/10.1016/S2542-5196(21)00251-5
2. Trewern, J., Chenoweth, J., Christie, I. and Halevy, S., 'Does promoting plant-based products in Veganuary lead to increased sales, and a reduction in meat sales? A natural experiment in a supermarket setting', *Public Health Nutrition* 25(11) (2022): https://doi.org/10.1017/S1368980022001914

3. Webb, A.R., Kazantzidis, A., Kift, R.C., et al., 'Meeting vitamin D requirements in white Caucasians at UK latitudes: providing a choice', *Nutrients* 10(4) (2018): https://doi.org/10.3390/nu10040497
4. Webb, A.R., Kazantzidis, A., Kift, R.C., et al., 'Colour counts: sunlight and skin type as drivers of vitamin D deficiency at UK latitudes', *Nutrients* 10(4) (2018), p. 457: https://doi.org/10.3390/nu10040457
5. NHS, 'Iron': https://www.nhs.uk/conditions/vitamins-and-minerals/iron/
6. Nagra, M., Tsam, F., Ward, S. and Ur, E., 'Animal vs plant-based meat: a hearty debate', *Canadian Journal of Cardiology* 40(7) (2024): https://doi.org/10.1016/j.cjca.2023.11.005
7. Hamlett, C., 'Is processed vegan food bad for your heart? A fact check', Plant Based News (19 June 2024): https://plantbasednews.org/lifestyle/health-and-fitness/is-processed-vegan-food-bad-for-your-heart-a-fact-check/
8. Whittaker, R. and Pickles, K., 'Vegan fake meats are linked to increase in heart deaths, study suggests: experts say plant-based diets can boost health – but NOT if they are ultra-processed', *Daily Mail* (10 June 2024): https://www.dailymail.co.uk/health/article-13513957/Plant-based-ultra-processed-foods-heart-death.html
9. Blackett, J., 'Vegans are slowly killing themselves', *Daily Telegraph* (11 June 2024): https://www.telegraph.co.uk/news/2024/06/11/vegans-are-slowly-killing-themselves-processed-food/
10. Farvid, Maryam S et al. 'Consumption of red meat and processed meat and cancer incidence: a systematic review and meta-analysis of prospective studies.' *European journal of epidemiology* vol. 36,9 (2021): 937-951. doi:10.1007/s10654-021-00741-9
11. Darmiento, L., 'How Beyond Meat is trying to get its sizzle back', *Los Angeles Times* (31 May 2024): https://www.latimes.com/business/story/2024-05-31/how-beyond-meat-lost-some-of-its-sizzle
12. Anderson, D.M., Brydon, W.G. and Eastwood, M.A., 'The dietary effects of gellan gum in humans', *Food Additives and Contaminants* 5(3) (1988): https://doi.org/10.1080/02652038809373701
13. *Veganuary 2024 Six Month Survey*, Veganuary: https://veganuary.com/wp-content/uploads/2024/09/Veganuary-2024-6-Month-Survey.pdf

CHAPTER 4: BEYOND FOOD

1. *Fur Trade in the UK: Seventh Report of Session 2017– 19,* Environment, Food and Rural Affairs Committee (2018): https://publications.parliament.uk/pa/cm201719/cmselect/cmenvfru/823/823.pdf
2. Bijleveld, M., *Natural Mink Fur and Faux Fur Products, an Environmental Comparison*, CE Delft (2013): https://cedelft.eu/publications/natural-mink-fur-and-faux-fur-products-an-environmental-comparison/

3. Hakansson, E., Carter, N., Coen, L. and LaBarbera, N., *Under Their Skin: Leather's Impact on the Planet*, Faunalytics (2022): https://static1.squarespace.com/static/5f5f02dd9b510014eef4fc4f/t/64025b58f16f565c702635cf/1677876106157/Leather%27s+impact+on+the+planet+report.pdf
4. Honan, K., 'Northern Co-operative Meat Company shoulders a $7 million loss after a challenging year', ABC News (17 December 2018): https://www.abc.net.au/news/rural/2018-12-17/casino-meatworks-reports-multimillion-dollar-loss/10620072
5. United Nations Industrial Development Organization, *Leather Carbon Footprint: Review of the European Standard EN 16887:2017* (2017): https://leatherpanel.org/sites/default/files/publications-attachments/leather_carbon_footprint_p.pdf
6. Ibid.
7. Hakansson, E., 'The carbon cost of our leather goods, calculated', Collective Fashion Justice: https://www.collectivefashionjustice.org/articles/carbon-cost-leather-goods
8. United Nations Industrial Development Organization, op. cit.
9. Laurenti, R., Redwood, M., Puig, R. and Frostell, B., 'Measuring the environmental footprint of leather processing technologies', *Journal of Industrial Ecology* 21(5) (2016): https://doi.org/10.1111/jiec.12504
10. Grant, H., 'Secret videos reveal workers beating sheep on English and Scottish farms', *Guardian* (16 November 2018): https://www.theguardian.com/environment/2018/nov/16/secret-videos-reveal-workers-beating-sheep-on-english-and-scottish-farms
11. Milman, O., 'Sheep cruelty video sparks RSPCA investigation', *Guardian* (11 July 2014): https://www.theguardian.com/world/2014/jul/11/sheep-cruelty-video-sparks-rspca-investigation
12. 'Shearing shed sheep cruelty footage "very concerning" – MPI', RNZ (17 January 2025): https://www.rnz.co.nz/news/national/539268/shearing-shed-sheep-cruelty-footage-very-concerning-mpi
13. Schmutz, M., Hischier, R. and Som, C., 'Factors allowing users to influence the environmental performance of their T-shirt', *Sustainability* 13(5) (2021): https://doi.org/10.3390/su13052498
14. Feldstein, S., Hakansson, E., Katcher, J. and Vance, U., *Shear Destruction: Wool, Fashion and the Biodiversity Crisis*, Center for Biological Diversity and Collective Fashion Justice's CIRCUMFAUNA Initiative (2021): https://static1.squarespace.com/static/5f5f02dd9b510014eef4fc4f/t/61afe2a0d31f175170d9a073/1638916793624/Shear+Destruction.pdf
15. Circumfauna, 'How do wool, lyocell and cotton knitwear compare, when it comes to land impact?': https://circumfauna.org/fibre-land-comparisons
16. Ibid.

NOTES

17. Poore, J. and Nemecek, T., 'Reducing food's environmental impacts through producers and consumers', *Science* 360(6392) (2018): https://www.science.org/doi/10.1126/science.aaq0216
18. Collective Fashion Justice, 'Issues in the down supply chain': https://www.collectivefashionjustice.org/down
19. Astudillo, M.F., Thalwitz, G. and Vollrath, F., 'Life cycle assessment of silk production – a case study from India' in S.S. Muthu (ed.), *Handbook of Life Cycle Assessment (LCA) of Textiles and Clothing* (Woodhead Publishing, 2016): https://doi.org/10.1016/B978-0-08-100169-1.00011-3
20. Hogeboom, R.J. and Hoekstra, A.Y., 'Water and land footprints and economic productivity as factors in local crop choice: the case of silk in Malawi', *Water* 9(10) (2017): https://doi.org/10.3390/w9100802
21. Vaughan, A., 'Man pours beer over tiger as London zoo Lates parties get out of hand', *Guardian* (18 July 2014): https://www.theguardian.com/environment/2014/jul/18/london-zoo-party-night-animal-welfare
22. Croucher, S., 'Elephants forced to perform underwater tricks in zoo: "Enough is enough"', Newsweek (9 October 2018): https://www.newsweek.com/elephant-zoo-forced-tricksunderwater-video-1159919
23. Animal Equality, *Caged Lives: An Animal Equality Undercover Investigation into Spanish Zoos* (2011): https://www.zoocheck.com/wp-content/uploads/2015/06/Spanish_Zoos_2011.pdf
24. Lindsay, M., 'Zoo faces animal welfare and bullying allegations', BBC News (16 October 2024): https://www.bbc.com/news/articles/cyvy96qd7p7o
25. Toliver, Z., 'European zoo authority agrees to add elephant protections – in 10 years?', PETA (23 July 2019): https://www.peta.org/blog/hanover-zoo-staff-caught-beating-baby-elephants-make-tricks/
26. Braitman, L., 'Even the gorillas and bears in our zoos are hooked on Prozac', *Wired* (15 July 2014): https://www.wired.com/2014/07/animal-madness-laurel-braitman/
27. Marris, E., 'Modern zoos are not worth the moral cost', *New York Times* (11 June 2011): https://www.nytimes.com/2021/06/11/opinion/zoos-animal-cruelty.html
28. Rawlinson, K., 'Rain-lashed penguins at Scarborough sanctuary given antidepressants', *Guardian* (6 February 2014): https://www.theguardian.com/world/the-northerner/2014/feb/06/penguins-prescribed-antidepressants-scarborough-rain
29. Smith, L., 'Zoos drive animals crazy', Slate (20 June 2014): https://slate.com/technology/2014/06/animal-madness-zoochosis-stereotypic-behavior-and-problems-with-zoos.html
30. Clubb, R., Rowcliffe, M., Lee, P., Mar, K.U. and Mason, G.J., 'Compromised survivorship in zoo elephants', *Science* 322(5908) (2008): https://www.science.org/doi/abs/10.1126/science.1164298

31. Born Free, *Elephants in Zoos: A Legacy of Shame* (2012): https://www.bornfree.org.uk/resource/elephants-in-zoos-a-legacy-of-shame/
32. British and Irish Association of Zoos and Aquariums, *BIAZA Animal Transfer Policy* (2023): https://biaza.org.uk
33. Fravel, L., 'Critics question zoos' commitment to conservation', *National Geographic* (13 November 2003): https://www.nationalgeographic.com/animals/article/news-zoo-commitment-conservation-critic
34. Brichieri-Colombi, T.A., Lloyd, N.A., McPherson, J.M., Moehrenschlager, A., 'Limited contributions of released animals from zoos to North American conservation translocations', *Conservation Biology* 33(1) (2019), pp.33–39: https://doi.org/10.1111/cobi.13160
35. Aspinal, D., 'Zooality check: the great zoo con' (2020): https://assets.publishing.service.gov.uk/media/61388969e90e07043b46127b/FOI2021_10084_Annex_I.pdf
36. Fernandez, C. and Keogh, G., 'London Zoo lion family is so inbred that two out of three cubs are dying: pride are all descended from small group of "founders" that shared the same grandparents', *Daily Mail* (27 December 2017): www.dailymail.co.uk/news/article-5216207/London-Zoo-lions-inbred-two-three-cubs-dying.html
37. Gilbert, T., Gardner, R., Kraaijeveld, A.R. and Riordan, P., 'Contributions of zoos and aquariums to reintroductions: historical reintroduction efforts in the context of changing conservation perspectives', *International Zoo Yearbook* 51(1) (2017): https://zslpublications.onlinelibrary.wiley.com/doi/abs/10.1111/izy.12159
38. BIAZA: https://biaza.org.uk/
39. BIAZA, 'Conserve': https://biaza.org.uk/conserve
40. Born Free, *Zoos: Financing Conservation or Funding Captivity?* (2021): https://www.bornfree.org.uk/resource/zoos-financing-conservation-or-funding-captivity/
41. Bekhechi, M., 'If you're really saddened by the death of Marius the giraffe, stop visiting zoos', *Independent* (10 February 2014): https://www.independent.co.uk/voices/comment/if-you-re-really-saddened-by-the-death-of-marius-the-giraffe-stop-visiting-zoos-9119868.html
42. Born Free, *Zoos* (2021)
43. 'Chester Zoo sees revenues rise 13% to £57.4m', *Liverpool Business News* (16 June 2024): https://lbndaily.co.uk/chester-zoo-sees-revenues-rise-13-to-57-4m/
44. Republic of Kenya, Office of the Auditor-General, *Report of the Auditor-General on Kenya Wildlife Service for the Year Ended 30 June, 2022* (2022): https://www.treasury.go.ke/wp-content/uploads/2024/10/Kenya-Wildlife-Service-2021_2022.pdf
45. Marino, L., Lilienfeld, S.O., Malamud, R., Nobis, N. and Broglio, R., 'Do zoos and aquariums promote attitude change in visitors? A critical

evaluation of the American zoo and aquarium study', *Society and Animals* 18(2) (2010): https://doi.org/10.1163/156853010X491980
46. Ibbetson, C., 'Where do Britons stand on animal testing?' YouGov (17 November 2021): https://yougov.co.uk/health/articles/39468-where-do-britons-stand-animal-testing

CHAPTER 5: NOW YOU'RE VEGAN, WHAT NEXT?

1. Association of UK Dieticians, 'Vegetarian, vegan and plant-based diet': https://www.bda.uk.com/resource/vegetarian-vegan-plant-based-diet.html
2. NHS, 'The vegan diet': https://www.nhs.uk/live-well/eat-well/how-to-eat-a-balanced-diet/the-vegan-diet/
3. Drake, M., 'Vegan couple who fed children only raw fruit and veg charged with murder after baby dies from starvation', *Independent* (20 December 2019): https://www.independent.co.uk/news/world/americas/vegan-couple-murder-baby-starve-ryan-patrick-o-leary-sheila-florida-a9255046.html
4. Mars, *United Kingdom State of Pet Homelessness Project* (2024): https://cms.stateofpethomelessness.com/s3media/2024-01/SoPH-United-Kingdom_0.pdf?VersionId=f3Jg0dd5XJ8NtTRc8su1TPpX2MNWc9Oy
5. The Charity Commission, 'Battersea Dogs' and Cats' Home annual report and consolidated financial statements: year ended 31 December 2023' (2023): https://shorturl.at/JxBDM
6. Gayle, D., 'Vets ask prospective dog owners to avoid pugs and other flat-faced breeds', *Guardian* (21 September 2016): https://www.theguardian.com/lifeandstyle/2016/sep/21/vets-ask-prospective-dog-owners-to-avoid-pugs-and-other-flat-faced-breeds
7. Wood, Z., 'Number of abandoned cats soars by more than 30% in UK', *Guardian* (23 October 2024): https://www.theguardian.com/world/2024/oct/23/number-of-abandoned-cats-soars-by-more-than-30-in-uk
8. Clark, A., 'The heartbreaking story of how animals are bred for the European pet trade', PETA UK (27 April 2015): https://www.peta.org.uk/blog/animals-breeders-european-pet-trade/
9. Okin, G.S., 'Environmental impacts of food consumption by dogs and cats', *PLoS ONE* 12(8) (2017): https://doi.org/10.1371/journal.pone.0181301
10. Newsround, 'Study analyses environmental impacts of pet diets', BBC (21 November 2022): https://www.bbc.co.uk/newsround/63673611
11. Okin, op. cit.
12. Alexander, P., Berri, A., Moran, D., Reay, D. and Rounsevell, M.D.A., 'The global environmental paw print of pet food', *Global Environmental Change* 65 (2020): https://doi.org/10.1016/j.gloenvcha.2020.102153
13. Meeker, D.L. and Meisinger, J.L., 'COMPANION ANIMALS SYMPOSIUM: Rendered ingredients significantly influence sustainability,

quality, and safety of pet food', *Journal of Animal Science* 93(3) (2015): https://doi.org/10.2527/jas.2014-8524
14. 'BVA policy position on diet choices for cats and dogs', British Veterinary Association (2024): https://www.bva.co.uk/media/5997/bva-policy-position-on-diet-choices-for-cats-and-dogs.pdf
15. Knight, A., Bauer, A. and Brown, H.J., 'Vegan versus meat-based dog food: guardian-reported health outcomes in 2,536 dogs, after controlling for canine demographic factors', *Heliyon* 10(17) (2024): https://doi.org/10.1016/j.heliyon.2024.e35578
16. Domínguez-Oliva, A., Mota-Rojas, D., Semendric, I. and Whittaker, A.L., 'The impact of vegan diets on indicators of health in dogs and cats: a systematic review', *Veterinary Sciences* 10(1) (2023): https://doi.org/10.3390/vetsci10010052
17. Kaindama, L., Jenkins, C., Aird, H., et al., 'A cluster of Shiga Toxin-producing *Escherichia coli* O157:H7 highlights raw pet food as an emerging potential source of infection in humans', *Epidemiology & Infection* 149 (2021): https://doi.org/10.1017/S0950268821001072
18. Sealey, J.E., Astley, B., Rollings, K. and Avison, M.B., 'Antibiotic resistant *Escherichia coli* in uncooked meat purchased from large chain grocery stores and in raw dog food purchased from pet stores in the same city', bioRxiv (2024): https://doi.org/10.1101/2024.03.03.583175
19. O'Halloran, C., Ioannidi, O., Reed, N., et al., 'Tuberculosis due to *Mycobacterium bovis* in pet cats associated with feeding a commercial raw food diet', *Journal of Feline Medicine and Surgery* 21(8) (2019): https://doi.org/10.1177/1098612X19848455
20. O'Halloran, C., Tørnqvist-Johnsen, C., Woods, G., et al., 'Feline tuberculosis caused by *Mycobacterium bovis* infection of domestic UK cats associated with feeding a commercial raw food diet', *Transboundary and Emerging Diseases* 68(4) (2021): https://doi.org/10.1111/tbed.13889
21. UK Pet Food, 'Vegetarian and vegan diets for cats and dogs' (November 2022): https://sustainablepetfoodassociation.co.uk/wp-content/uploads/2023/01/Vegetarian-and-vegan-Diets-2022-Nov.pdf
22. Davies, M., Alborough, R., Jones, L., et al., 'Mineral analysis of complete dog and cat foods in the UK and compliance with European guidelines', *Scientific Reports* 7 (2017): https://doi.org/10.1038/s41598-017-17159-7

CHAPTER 6: HOW TO BE VEGAN IN A NON-VEGAN WORLD

1. Willett, W., Rockström, J., Loken, B., Springmann, M. and Lang, T., 'Food in the Anthropocene: the EAT-*Lancet* Commission on healthy diets from sustainable food systems', *The Lancet* 393(10170) (2019): https://doi.org/10.1016/S0140-6736(18)31788-4
2. Carlile, C., 'Revealed: meat industry behind attacks on flagship climate-friendly diet report', DeSmog (10 April 2025): https://www.desmog.

com/2025/04/10/meat-industry-red-flag-animal-agriculture-alliance-behind-attacks-flagship-climate-friendly-diet-report-eat-lancet/
3. Carlile, C., 'PR campaign may have fuelled food study backlash, leaked document shows', *Guardian* (11 April 2025): https://www.theguardian.com/environment/2025/apr/11/pr-campaign-may-fuelled-food-study-backlash-leaked-document-eat-lancet
4. Ritchie, H., 'You want to reduce the carbon footprint of your food? Focus on what you eat, not whether your food is local', Our World in Data (24 January 2020): https://ourworldindata.org/food-choice-vs-eating-local

ACKNOWLEDGEMENTS

Each of the three books that I've written so far have been different experiences for me, and each has formed key memories that have punctuated periods of my life and my work. Yet one thing that has remained constant throughout the writing process for each book is the support I have received and the places that support has come from.

With this in mind, I want to express my deep gratitude and appreciation to Penguin Random House and the team at Ebury for our third collaboration. A special thank you to Sam Jackson, who has been the person behind each of these three collaborations and to whom I owe a great deal of gratitude. A huge thank you as well to Sonam Nundoochan, Aisling O'Toole, Jasleen Dhindsa, and everyone else at Ebury for their work and time on this book.

One of the things I enjoy most about writing is the commitment that it requires and the dedicated time that has to be put towards it; however, that commitment and time also mean it requires trust and belief from everyone else involved in the process. So, rather than my gratitude simply being for the opportunity to write another book, I am also deeply appreciative of the trust and belief that those who gave me this opportunity have afforded me.

Thank you again to Paul Murphy. It's been a pleasure collaborating with you for the third time, and I appreciate your insights and thoughtful scrutiny of my writing, arguments and ideas. Thank you also to Jordan Lees, Hattie Grunewald and The Blair Partnership for believing in me as an author and for supporting me and my ideas.

An extra special thank you goes to my wife, just as it has for the previous books too. Thank you for always supporting me and for all of your work behind the scenes. An honourable mention must also go to all of the delicious breakfasts of oatmeal with berries, flaxseed and nut butter that you made for me. They were both delicious and the ideal way to start a day of writing.

I would also like to acknowledge all of you who have supported my work throughout the years. While I am extremely grateful for the opportunities I have had, I have only had the privilege to be able to spend time advocating for veganism because of the support I have received. So thank you so much for all of the trust, kindness and generosity that you have offered me throughout the years. The reason I have been able to write this book – and the ones before it – is because of all of you. My deepest gratitude to each and every one of you.

And finally, to those of you who have read this book because you're interested in going vegan, thank you for reading this book and thank you for considering veganism. I really hope that you've found value in this book and that it helps you go (and stay) vegan.

INDEX

acceptance 200–5
advertising 197–9, 204, 214–18
advocacy 171–2, 174, 211–12
Albanese, Anthony 215–16
albumen 88
alcohol consumption 94–6
algal blooms 30
algal oil supplements 104
almonds 101, 115, 118, 213
alpha-linolenic acid (ALA) 104, 115
amino acids, essential 101
anaemia 100
animal abuse 12, 22, 64, 136, 151–2, 183, 201
Animal Agriculture Alliance 214–15
animal appreciation 218–20
animal cruelty 12–13, 31–2, 64, 129, 136, 151–2, 196
  see also cruelty-free brands
animal exploitation 7–8, 11–16, 61, 67, 127–8, 142, 196, 200, 209–10, 220–3
  and animal family separation 216
  and animal testing 159–61
  and Burger King 92
  and cell-cultured meat 111–13
  and children 180
  and clothing 128, 137, 142
  and entertainment 148–9, 151–2, 157
  hiding the truth about 40
  ignorance surrounding 198

and 'may contain' products 90
and pandemics 19–20, 22
and pets 183, 191
scale 11, 32
wildlife 19, 20
animal family separation 13, 216
animal farming 7–8, 197, 198
  and antibiotic use 17–19
  and deforestation 21, 27, 28, 61
  disconnecting from cruelty 42
  environmental impact 7–8, 25–7, 57, 61, 213–14
  and fur 129–30
  and habitat loss 21, 27, 30
  hiding the truth about 40
  and pandemics 19–22
  and pet food 187
  secretive nature 218
  and supplements 105
  unnatural nature 112
  and wool 138
animal feed 30–1, 61, 186–93
animal forcible impregnation 12, 13, 14
animal mutilation 12, 14, 152, 200
animal products 70–2, 204, 216–18
  clothing 12, 13, 128–47, 176
  and cruelty-free products 160
  marketing/advertising 197–9, 204, 214–18
  medicines 162–3
  see also specific products

animal products (foods) 13, 31, 38–42, 82
  and baking 114
  and balanced diets 100
  and children 178–9, 181
  cross-contamination 89–92
  disconnecting from cruel processes 40–2
  and food labels 85–93
  and health 79
  as hidden ingredients 85–93
  iron content 103
  marketing/advertising 197–9
  negative impact 11
  and non-vegan partners 175
  and perspectives 38–40
  price 83–5
  protein 66
  waste/left-over 93–4
  see also specific products
animal sanctuaries 71–2, 158
animal shelters 183, 185
animal sterilisation 185–6
animal suffering 12, 15, 16, 90, 129, 157, 184, 190, 195–6, 199, 204, 209
animal testing 12, 13, 159–61, 162
animal welfare 3, 8, 217–18
animal-to-human transmission 20, 22
antibiotics 139
  and fish farms 30
  as growth promoters 17–18
  prophylactic 17, 18
  resistance 8–9, 16–19, 188
aquaculture 30
aquafaba 95, 114
aquariums 12, 127–8, 148–9, 155–7, 175, 208

bacteria 9, 15–16, 18, 188, 191
Bailey's 94
baking 114
balance 205–7
balanced diets 100, 115

bamboo 140
Barnivore 96
beans 78, 84, 98, 101, 103, 117–19
bears 149, 152, 153
bedding 140
beef 29, 82–3, 131–2, 190
beer 94–6
bees 88
behavioural change 35–67, 210, 224
  making 1–5, 7–33
behavioural disruption 36
Benchley, Peter 148
Beyond Meat 109
biodiversity 27–8, 31, 155
biomass 28, 30
bioreactors 112–13
bird flu 15, 20, 139
birthday parties 180–1
Blackfish (2013) 148
blood tests 106, 167
blowflies 136
body language 64
bolt guns 12
boundary-setting 169, 171, 173–5
bowel movements 97
breakfasts 115–17
breeders 183–4
breeding, selective 136–7, 140, 184, 191
breeding programs 153–5
British Dietic Association 106, 176, 213
buckwheat 101, 120
Buddha bowls 118
bullfighting 149, 208
burger alternatives 109, 121
Burger King 90, 91–3
bushmeat 22
butcher's shops 203–6
by-products 187, 190–1

cages 12, 129, 158–9
calcium 56, 101–2, 109–10, 178
calories 98–9
campylobacter 22

INDEX

cancer 16, 23–4, 102, 108
carbon cycle 29
carbon dioxide
   emissions 26, 28
   storage/sequestration 28–9, 31
carbon sinks 29
cardiovascular health 107–8
carmine 89, 160
carnivores, obligate 189
cars 146–7
casein 87
casseroles 120–1
castration 135
cats 64, 183, 186–93, 219–20
   meat trade 11, 15, 39, 78, 183
Cats Protection 185
cattle 13, 61, 71, 131–2, 213, 216
   see also cows
cell-cultured meat 111–13, 142, 193, 208
change 35–67, 210, 224
   making the 1–5, 7–33
cheese 2, 38, 41, 52, 79, 90, 98
   vegan 77, 79–84, 110, 117–19, 170
Chester Zoo 156–7
chia seed pudding 116
chickens 15, 29, 31–2, 71, 83, 158, 188, 195
chickpea water 95
chickpeas 117
children 176–82
China 134–5, 139
choice 31–2, 38–9
chromium 131, 134
chronic disease 8, 22–5, 79, 97, 103
circuses 12, 149, 150, 151
cleaning products 159–61, 171
climate catastrophe 25, 214
climate change 20, 22, 25–6, 29, 31–2
clothing 12, 13, 128–47, 176
cochineal 89
cocktails 95
coffee 87

cognitive behavioural therapy (CBT) 203, 207
cognitive biases 35, 48
cognitive dissonance 62
communication skills 60–5
communities, like-minded 67–9, 92
conservation 153, 155–7
cooking 44–5, 113–22, 125, 170–1
Copenhagen Zoo 154
cosmetics 88, 89, 127, 159–61
cotton 131, 138, 140–1
Covid-19 pandemic 21, 185
cows 13, 17, 64, 132, 158, 190, 195
cows' milk 39, 43, 83, 102
   alternatives 43, 66, 81–3, 87, 102, 109–10, 115–17, 221
   on food labels 87
   as ingredient 46, 86, 87, 94, 108, 160
crisps 46
crops, land use 27, 28
cross-contamination 89–92
cruelty-free brands 127, 159–61, 171
crustaceans 87
culling 21
cultural norms 9, 36, 39, 57, 75, 124, 179, 188, 221, 221–2, 222
curries 44, 120

dairy 29, 57, 65
   and cruelty 13
   cutting out 53
   environmental impact 214
   and food labels 87
   see also cheese; Cows' milk
dairy alternatives 77, 79–84, 102, 109–10, 117–19, 170
   see also plant-based milk
dairy industry 13, 17, 51–2, 132, 216
dairy-free 77, 87
dating 172–4, 223
De Laurentiis, Dino 148
deforestation 21, 27–8, 61, 135

deprivation 222–3
desserts 114
diabetes 108
digestive enhancers 17–18
dinners 119–21
disease 19–22, 30
  see also chronic disease; pandemics
disinformation 212–15
docosahexaenoic acid (DHA) 104, 105
dogs 12, 64, 183–9, 192, 203
  meat trade 11, 15, 78, 183
dolphins 39, 78, 128, 149, 153
down 139–40
ducks 139, 203, 204

E. coli 22, 188
E-numbers 89
Eat-*Lancet* report 214–15
eating out 87, 90–3, 122–3, 173–4
Ebola 22
ecosystems 27, 29, 31
education 10
eggs 13, 51–2, 57, 65
  alternatives 77
  cutting out 53
  egg white 88, 95
  environmental impact 214
  and food labels 87
  as source of vitamin D 102
eicosapentaenoic acid (EPA) 104, 105
electrocution 12, 129
elephants 151, 152–3, 153
emissions 25–9, 31, 133–4, 138, 187
emotional side of veganism 71, 200–7, 220
emotional wellbeing 37
empathy 39, 71
endangered animals 153–5
enteric fermentation 26
entertainment, use of animals for 12–13, 147–59
environmental concerns 3, 8–9, 25–32, 210, 213–14
  see also emissions; land use; sustainability
ethical veganism 7
ethics 7–9, 11–16, 31–2, 37, 57, 61–2, 64, 210, 216–18, 222
  and animal farming 198
  and cell-cultured meat 111
  and children 181
  and clothing 132–3, 135, 137, 142, 144
  and cosmetics/cleaning products 159
  of how we treat animals 8, 9
  and leather 132–3
  and meat 216
  and medication 161–2
  and pets 183, 190, 193
  and rodeos 146
euthanasia 183
experimentation 12, 13, 159–61, 162
exposés 15
extinction 155

families, non-vegan 53–68, 65–7, 70, 72–3, 169, 199–200, 220
farmable land, infertile 22
farming
  intensive 17, 19–20, 139, 217
  see also animal farming
fashion industry 142
  see also clothing
feather plucking 12
fertiliser 26–7
fibre 97
fish 12, 31–2, 104, 217
  consumption levels 11
  and food labels 87
  oily 102
  pets' consumption of 187, 190, 192
  swim bladders 95–6
  see also pescatarian diets
fish oil 104
fishing 28–31, 208

INDEX

fishmongers 217
fluoroquinolones 188
flystrike 136
foetal bovine serum 111
foie gras 139
food
  navigating as a vegan 75–125
  supply 20
  what to eat 76–96
  see also animal products (food); *specific foods*
food allergens 87, 89–90, 95
food chains 29
food cravings 45, 46–51
food labels 85–93
food security 25
formula milk 178
fortified foods 102, 104–5, 107, 110, 117, 189
friends, non-vegan 53–67, 70, 72–3, 169–72, 220, 223
fur 12, 129–31, 144

gains of veganism 37, 79, 96–8, 106
gas chambers 12, 13, 15, 127, 129, 140, 196, 199–200, 204
geese 139
gelatine 88, 162–3
gellan gum 109–10
generalisations 48
giraffes 154
global problems 9
global warming 213
goal-setting, achievable 50, 53
gorillas 152, 156
grazing 13, 27, 28, 46, 213, 218
greenhouse gases 25–9, 31, 138, 187
growth promoters 17–18
guilt 14, 39, 47, 48, 209, 212
guinea pigs 40

habitat loss 21, 27, 30
habitats, marine 29
habits, new 36–7
Happy Cow website/app 122–3

harm 12, 27, 30, 40, 57, 67, 97, 102, 107, 137, 144, 147, 157, 169–70, 183, 190–1, 196, 216, 221, 222
health
  and the benefits of plant-based eating 79, 96–8, 106
  concerns 55–6
  and healthy eating 1, 46, 55–6, 98–110, 106
  holistic approach to 106, 166
high-income countries 31
hippos, pygmy 151–2
honey 88, 94
horses 49
hostility, dealing with 56–61, 72–3
hot dog alternatives 121
human immunodeficiency virus (HIV) 22
human-to-human transmission 20
hunger 45–6, 99
hunters/hunting 129, 215–16
hypertension 108
hypocrisy 61–2, 92, 146, 215

identity 75, 210–12
ignorance 10, 197–9
intellectual veganism 71
iodine 105, 178
iron, dietary 56, 103–4, 107, 109, 167, 178
  deficiency 168
isinglass 95–6
isolation 67, 69

Jaws (1975) 148
Jones, Sam 215–16

Kenya Wildlife Service 157
knowledge, power of 32–3

lac beetles 89
lactose 87, 95, 163
lactose-free 87
lamb 29, 135–6

lambs 190, 216
land use 27–8, 31
landfill 133
language, use of 64
lanolin 88, 160
leading by example 171–2, 174
'Leaping Bunny' logo 159, 160
leather 128, 131–5, 138, 142, 143, 144–7
  as by-product 131–2, 134
  synthetic 133–4, 142, 145–6
left-over food 93–4
legumes 23, 77, 78, 95, 99, 101, 110, 115, 120
lions 149–50, 153–5, 158–9
listening skills 63
living arrangements,
  with non-vegans 169–72, 174–6, 180, 199–201, 223
local food 217, 218
London Zoo 150–1, 155, 156
low-sugar diets 42–3
lunches 117–19
lyocell 138, 141

'macerated alive' 12, 13, 15
malnutrition 176–7
mangroves 29
manure 26, 27
marine ecosystems 29, 31
Marius (giraffe) 154
marketing 197–9, 204, 214–18
mastitis 17
'may contain' label 89–93
McDonald's 92–3
meal plans 46, 114
meals, plant-based 44, 113–22
meat 2, 13, 22–3, 32, 38–42, 47, 57, 63, 65, 98, 103, 108, 199, 204, 208
  as cultural norm 57
  cutting out 53
  disconnecting from cruel processes 40–2
  environmental impact 214
  and ethics 216
  global demand for 19–20, 25
  and health 107
  pets' consumption of 186–93
  preferences 79
  social pressure to eat 67
  sustainability 31–2, 216
  unconventional 11, 15, 39, 78
  see also cell-cultured meat; red meat
meat alternatives 66, 76–7, 80, 82–3, 85, 101, 107–9, 110, 117–20, 121
meat markets 22
medication 161–3
menstruation 103
methane emissions 26, 28
milk see cows' milk; formula milk; plant-based milk
milk powder 46, 86
milk-derived products 163
  see also lactose
mince, plant-based 85
mindfulness 203
misinformation 212–15
molluscs 87
Moo Deng (pygmy hippo) 151–2
mulberry 141
mulesing 136
Musk, Elon 213–14

National Health Service (NHS) 106, 176, 213
natural resources 19
natural world, degradation 25
'new normal' 35–73
Nipah 22
nitrous oxide emissions 26
nut butters 99, 115
nutrients 99–106, 167
nutritional deficiencies 100, 165–9
nuts 99

oat milk 87
oats, over-night 115–16
oceans 29

omega-3 fatty acids 56, 104, 115
orcas 148, 159

pandemics 8, 9, 19–22, 185
partners
    non-vegan 174–6, 180, 201
    see also dating
pasta 44, 119–20
peer pressure 67–70
penicillin 17
perspectives/perceptions 38–40, 205–7
pescatarian diets 84
pets 182–93, 203, 219, 223
photosynthesis 28
physical wellbeing 37
phytoplankton 29
pigeons 218–19, 220
piglets 216
pigs 13, 20, 64, 71, 158, 190, 196, 203, 205
plant-based diets 3–4, 7–8, 31–2, 75, 92–3, 125, 127
    alternatives 4, 65–6, 76–85, 101, 102, 107–11, 121, 170–1, 197
    for animals 30, 186–93
    and antibiotic resistance 19
    arguments for 7
    attacks on 214, 215
    and children 176–8, 180, 182
    and cross-contamination 90–2
    and eating out 122
    and emissions 26, 31
    and environmental considerations 26, 149–50
    and food labels 85–6, 90
    and greenhouse gas emissions 26
    and health 22–4, 79, 98–109, 166–9
    and hunger 46
    and land use 28
    making it your goal 50
    meals 44, 113–22
    misinformation surrounding 212–15
    and non-vegans 170–1, 175, 209
    not liking 79–83
    and nutritional deficiencies 166–9
    and pets 186–93
    price 83–5
    processed nature 107
    and protein 66, 100–1
    and sustainability 32
    talking to friends and family about 54, 55–6, 62–3, 65–6
    transitioning to 44, 50–1, 53
    and travelling 124
    what to expect on 96–7
plant-based milk 43, 66, 81–3, 87, 102, 109–10, 115–17
polyester 131, 137–8, 141
population growth 25
porridge 115
positivity 208–10
poultry 20
    see also chickens; ducks; geese
pride 14
processed food 76, 106–10
promoting veganism 171–2, 174, 211–12
propolis 88
protein 56
    complete 101
    meals 116, 118–20
    plant-based 66, 100–1
Przewalski's horse 153
psychological wellbeing 37
public-health threats 16
    see also antibiotics, resistance
pugs 184
puppy mills 186

quinoa 101, 117, 118, 120

rabbits 186, 193
rainforests 60–1
rats 219
raw-meat diets 188, 191
recipes 113–22
Red Flag 214–15

red meat 23, 38, 40–1, 53, 98, 103, 108, 138, 168, 214
reforestation 29
Responsibile Down Standard (RDS) 139
reward incentives 70–1
rewilding 28
rodents 21, 186, 219
rodeos 146, 149
Rogan, Joe 213–14
royal jelly 88
Royal Society for the Prevention of Cruelty to Animals (RSPCA) 185
ruminant animals 26
  see also cattle; cows; sheep

salads 76, 77, 118–19
salmonella 17–18, 22
sandwiches 117
SARS 22
satiety 99
sausages, plant-based 83, 101, 121
sea lions 148–9
seagrasses 29
second-hand clothing 143–7
seed butters 115
seed oils 213
seitan 66, 78, 101
selective abstraction 48
selective breeding 136–7, 140, 184, 191
selenium 105
self-compassion 48, 72
setbacks 73
shame 14, 47, 48
Shankly, Bill 221
sharks 147–8
sheep 71, 158
  see also lambs
shellac 89, 160
silk 140–1, 142
slaughter 11–14, 16, 31–2, 42, 137, 196, 199–200
  and cell-cultured meat 111
  and dairy animals 13
  and down 139
  and fur 129
  and hens 13
  and leather 132
  rates of 11
  see also culling; electrocution; gas chambers; maceration of living animals
slaughterhouses 13–15, 22, 40, 132–3, 196–7, 199, 218
smell, sense of 43
snacks 46
social conformity 67–70
social norms 222
  see also cultural norms
social pressure 67–70
soil degradation 28
soups 119
soya milk 83
soya products 61, 83, 101, 119
spicy food 43
Spielberg, Steven 148
squirrels 219
status quo bias 35
staying vegan, in a non-vegan world 4, 195–220
stews 120–1
stir-fries 120
Stoicism 201
STOPP technique 207
stress 166
sugar 42–3
sunlight 102–3
supermarkets 2, 39–41, 45, 66, 77, 84–5, 90, 92, 120, 123–4, 160, 178, 195, 197, 216, 221
supplements 102–3, 104–6, 167–9
sustainability 216–18
  clothing 132–4, 135, 138, 142, 144
  down 139
  fishing 29, 30–1
  food system 25, 29, 30–1, 213, 216
  leather 132–4

meat 216
pets 187, 193
wool 135, 138
swine flu 20
synthetic fabrics 137–8, 140–2

tail-docking 135
taste preferences 79–83
taste, sense of 42–3
tempeh 78, 101, 108, 118, 120
therapy 203, 205, 207
throat-cutting 13
tofu 2, 65–6, 78–9, 101, 103, 108, 116–20, 221
    scrambled tofu on sourdough bread 116
toiletries 159–61
traps 129
travel 123–4
tribes, finding your 67–9
tuberculosis, bovine 191

ultra-processed foods (UPFs) 106–10
United Nations (UN) 29
United Nations Environment Programme (UNEP) 19–20, 26
United Nations Industrial Development Organization (UNIDO) 133
urine 27

validation 63, 71
values 37, 64, 178–9, 181–2, 197, 216
vegan lifestyles
    advantages of 37, 79, 96–8, 106
    change of 1–5, 7–33, 35–67, 210, 224
    maintaining 4, 195–220
    navigation 165–93
Veganuary 125
Vegetarian Society 89

vegetarianism 13, 51–2, 85–6
venison 84–5
viruses 20–3, 139
vitamin B12 1, 56, 105, 107, 109, 178
    deficiency 100, 167
vitamin C 103
vitamin D 102–3, 104, 109, 110, 117, 178, 189
    D2 88
    D3 88, 103, 105
    deficiency 100

waste food 93–4
water intake 97
water pollution 31
water use 31
weight loss 98
welfare standards 197, 198
wellbeing 37
wellness industry 84
whales 78, 128
'whataboutery' 61–2
whey 87
wholegrains 99, 101, 118
wholewheat 119–20
wildlife 19, 20–2, 152–3
wildlife centres 158
wine 95–6
wombats 215–16
wool 135–9, 143, 144
    alternatives 137
    merino 136
World Health Organization (WHO) 16, 188
wraps 117

zoochosis 152
Zoological Society of London 155
zoonotic diseases 19–20
zoos 148–58, 175

ABOUT THE AUTHOR

On 14 May 2014, Ed Winters was reading the news online when the headline *Hundreds of chickens killed in M62 lorry crash* grabbed his attention. He clicked on the article and was stunned to read that about 1,500 chickens had been killed in a truck that had crashed while on the way to a slaughterhouse. This article became a huge catalyst in Ed's life, first encouraging him to go vegetarian before he eventually became vegan in 2015.

In early 2016, Ed set up his YouTube channel, where he began uploading street interviews with members of the public on the ethics of eating animals. In the same year, he also co-founded the animal rights organisation Surge, as well as The Official Animal Rights March, a global event which grew from 2,500 participants in London in 2016 to 41,000 participants across the world in 2019. Ed continues to be the co-director of Surge, with the organisation focusing on producing films that tell the untold stories of animals.

Just over a year after co-founding Surge, he released the documentary *Land of Hope and Glory*, which is an exposé of UK terrestrial animal farming. Ed then began touring UK universities to screen the documentary to students, where he also gave a speech to the students after the screening. His university speech *You Will Never Look at Your Life in the Same Way Again*, which has been given to thousands of students across UK universities, went viral in early 2018 and to date has 35 million accumulative views online.

Regularly lecturing on animal ethics and the environment, Ed has spoken at over one-third of UK universities and at every Ivy League college, including as a guest lecturer at Harvard University. He has given speeches across the world, including at LinkedIn, American Express, Pinterest, Google and Meta. Ed has additionally given three TEDx talks, surpassing a total of 2.6 million views online.

Ed has debated numerous times on live television and radio, and has been featured on the *BBC*, *ITV*, *LadBible* and *GB News*, and he has been featured by print and online news organisations including The *Guardian*, the *Independent* and *The Times*. In December 2020, Ed announced that he and his team had founded Surge Sanctuary, a forever home for abused and unwanted animals on an 18-acre site in rural England.

In 2021, Ed wrote his debut book *This is Vegan Propaganda (And Other Lies the Meat Industry Tells You)*, which was published by Penguin Random House on 6 January 2022, becoming an instant bestseller. In 2023, he published his second book *How to Argue With a Meat Eater (And Win Every Time)*, which was also published by Penguin Random House.

In 2022, Ed became a Media & Design Fellow at Harvard University, teaching a module during the fall semester. In 2023, he won a Webby People's Voice Award for his short film *Milk*. In 2025, Ed released the short film *Matilda and the Brave Escape*, which won multiple awards and was screened at film festivals around the world.

Also by Ed Winters

This is Vegan Propaganda

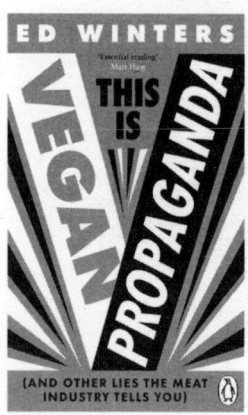

Every time we eat, we have the power to radically transform the world we live in.

Our choices can help alleviate the most pressing issues we face today: the climate crisis, infectious and chronic diseases, human exploitation and, of course, non-human exploitation. These issues can be uncomfortable to learn about but the benefits of doing so cannot be overstated. It is quite literally a matter of life and death.

Based on years of research and conversations with slaughterhouse workers, animal rights philosophers, environmentalists and everyday consumers, vegan educator Ed Winters answers the most pressing question, is there a better way?

This Is Vegan Propaganda is the empowering and groundbreaking book on veganism that everyone, vegan and sceptic alike, needs to read.

How to Argue with a Meateater

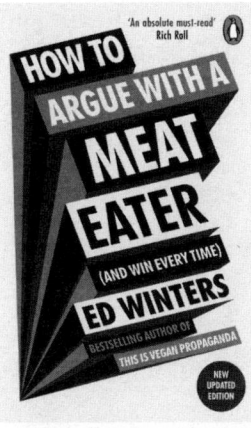

Challenge their beliefs; change the world

If you are a vegan, you'll know all too well how provocative it can be – you never know when you'll be challenged or how. But being able to face down and rebut arguments against veganism is hugely important. Not just because many of the arguments lack substance, but because every interaction provides a pivotal moment to create change.

How to Argue with a Meateater will teach you to not only become a skilled debater, but it will also arm you with powerful facts and insights that will give pause to even the most devout meat eater.

Providing you with the knowledge to become a better conversationalist and critical thinker, and the motivation to create a more ethical and sustainable world, let this book be your guide and inspiration to know that, no matter what the argument, you can win every time.